KABIR:
IN THE LIGHT OF KRIYAYOGA

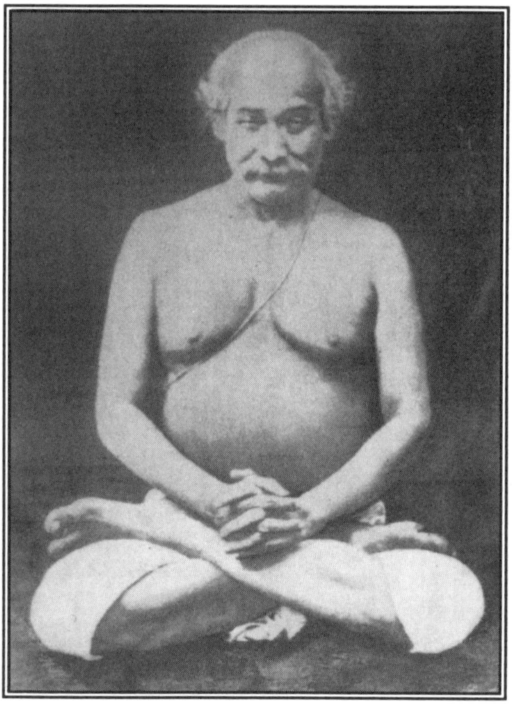

Yogiraj Shri Shri Shyama Charan Lahiri Mahashay
Advent: Ashwin 16, 1235 B.S. (1828 A.D.)
Mahasamadhi: Ashwin 10, 1302 B.S. (1895 A.D.)

KABIR
In the Light of Kriyayoga

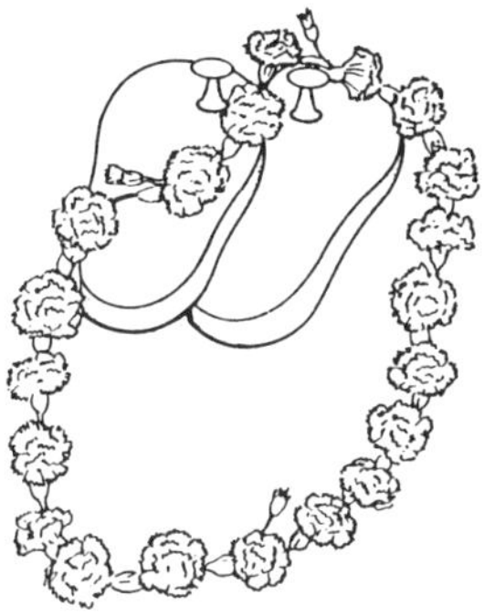

Translated and Edited

By

Prof. Jogesh Chandra Bhattacharya

M.A., P.R.S.

AMRITA FOUNDATION, INC.

Dallas, Texas

1997

Originally
Published in India with the First Edition in 1974
by Jogesh Chandra Bhattacharya, M.A., P.R.S.
at 'Shrigurudham' in Howrah.

ISBN: 0-937134-21-X

Printed in the United States of America

Amrita Foundation, Inc. is dedicated to the original Kriyayoga teachings of Shri Shri Lahiri Mahashay as given to him by Mahavatar Babaji, and the original, unchanged writings of Paramhansa (Swami) Yogananda Giri and Swami Dhirananda Giri (Dr. Basu Kumar Bagchi) to promote individual communion with God.
This First American Edition is a reprint of the First Edition published in India in 1974, with minor grammatical corrections.
The Publisher's Note and footnotes have been inserted.

The inside picture of Shri Shri Lahiri Mahashay is from the personal collection of Swami Dhirananda Giri (Dr. Basu Kumar Bagchi).

Published by

Amrita® FOUNDATION, INC

P.O. Box 190978
Dallas, Texas 75219-0978

To
The Lotus - Feet
of
My beloved Master
Yogiguru Shri Shri Thakur Anilanandaji Maharaj

Publisher's Note

Inscrutable are the ways of the Divine! Some 20 years ago one of Paramhansa Yogananda's dearest and most advanced American women disciples, Mary Buchanan ("Kamala" – the name bestowed on her by her Guru Yoganandaji at their first meeting in 1925) Silva, and her late husband, Edward J. Silva sent as a gift to Amrita Foundation a copy of this most profound book, *Kabir: In the Light of Kriyayoga* by J. C. Bhattacharya,who rendered it into English. The original book was written by one of Lahiri Mahashay's foremost direct disciples, Yogacharya Shrimat Panchanan Bhattacharya, founder of the now defunct Aryan Mission in Calcutta.

Well-known in India and because of its great value to the Kriya teachings, Kamala so deeply wanted then that Amrita Foundation publish the *Kabir* book for all devotees of our Kriyayoga Path. But since the publishing of such a book required additional funds and care in type setting, not only for the English translation, but also for the couplets of Kabir in the Hindi language, this most wonderful edition remained on the bookshelf for all these years . Until now – with the coming of Shibendu Lahiri, the Guru great grandson of Lahiri Mahashay who is spreading the Kriyas of Babaji and the Lahiri Lineage, auspiciously, funds and talent finally have come together to produce this most treasured volume on Kriyayoga.

Looking back on the events surrounding the journey of this sacred work into America, the book was sent to Kamala and Edward by devotees in Australia. There was one devotee in particular, who wishes to remain incognito, that was a devout Kriyaban in the Australian Meditation Group of Paramhansa Yoganandaji that made the English translation of the book possible through his enthusiastic and thoughtful spiritual support, as well as, his financial support. It was this devout Kriyaban, who was in correspondence at that time with J. C. Bhattacharya, and who commissioned him to translate the book into English. Mr. Bhattacharya, a renown scholar and follower of the Kriyayoga of Babaji and Lahiri Mahashay, was a great devotee of his Guru, Shri Shri Thakur Anilanandaji Maharaj, Preceptor of Shrigurudham (Yogada

Satsanga), Kadamtala Branch. It was Yogada Satsanga, established in 1919 at the Serampore Hermitage of Jnanavatar Shrimat Swami Yukteshwar by Yogishwar Shri Shri Matilal Thakur that Paramhansa Yogananda and his spiritual brother, Swami Dhirananda (Dr. Basu Kumar Bagchi) of Shri Yukteshwar's Puri Ashram also attended and received spiritual insights and instruction from.

Thus, the Leela of the Lord plays itself out in the world, linking Truth-seekers, one-to-another.

It is Amrita's blessed good fortune to publish this revered edition of sacred writings on our Kriya disciplines.

We joyfully offer *Kabir: In the Light of Kriyayoga* to the Lotus-Feet of Lahiri Mahashay and His Radiant Son, Shibendu Lahiri.

The Editor

June 25, 1997
Dallas, Texas

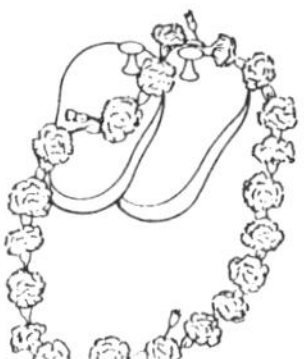

Shri Shri Gurabe Namah
Ohm

Preface

It is with the Grace of our beloved Master Shri Shri Thakur Anilanandaji Maharaj that the English version of Kabīr's 'dohā's or couplets is out at last.

Kabīr was a Muslim Saint in India born near Vārānasī (Benares) about 1440, A.D. He had his spiritual initiation in early life from the great Hindu sage Rāmānanda. The story of his life is an admixture of facts and legends. Some take him to be the son of a Hindu Brāhman adopted by a Muslim weaver at Benares. He was uneducated, and a family man who earned his living at the loom. Although he was persecuted in his life for mystic faith, he was later on held in the highest esteem by Hindus as well as Muslims. The legend goes that, after his death (in 1518), when his Hindu and Mohamedan disciples quarreled among themselves as to the mode of his funeral – cremation or burial – the figure of Kabīr appeared before them asking them to remove the winding sheet from the dead body. To their utter surprise they found on the coffin but a handful of flowers and not the body of the Saint. In the meantime the figure of Kabīr disappeared. The disciples of the two communities divided the flowers and the last rites were performed according to their different customs.

Kabīr composed hundreds of songs and couplets in popular Hindi of his times. Some of his songs have been translated into English by Rabindranath Tagore (Macmillan & Co. Limited, 1915).

Yogiraj Shri Shri Shyama Charan Lahiri Mahashay, the great reviver of Yoga in modern times, was very fond of the couplets of Kabīr breathing as they do great spiritual truths in symbolic language. The Yogiraj, as he did with many other religious books, showed the way to his disciples to interpret the deeper meanings of the Scriptures and the message of Saints in the light of Rājayoga or Kriyāyoga. Although he himself did not write these interpretations, one of his great disciples, Yogacharya Shrimat Panchanan Bhattacharya (Founder, the now defunct Arya Mission, Calcutta), was inspired to collect a few hundred couplets of Kabīr and interpret them in the light of his own Master.

The following is a humble attempt to present the same to the English reading public. It is however, not an exact translation. More often than not, the editor had to explain at much greater length the intention of the original, which, otherwise would have been unintelligible to the lay reader.

Our grateful thanks are due to the lovers and disciples of Paramhansa Yoganandaji Maharaj (dearest spiritual brother to Guru's Guru, Yogishwar Matilal Thakur Maharaj, Founder, Shrigurudham) in Australia. But for their inspiration and liberal donation the publication of this book would not probably have taken place at all. They, however, being true lovers of the Gurus and the Divine, like to remain incognito.

I should not also miss this opportunity to thank one of my highly respected spiritual brothers, Mr. Santosh Kumar Dey, Engineer, who has supplied all the requisite paper for printing this book during these days of paper crisis.

But after all, my beloved Guruji, Master Dearest, but for Your Grace and constant guidance, your humble disciple would never feel able to cope with the task. Let the fruit of this labor be offered to your Lotus Feet, Joy Guru.

Jogesh Chandra Bhattacharya

During 1974

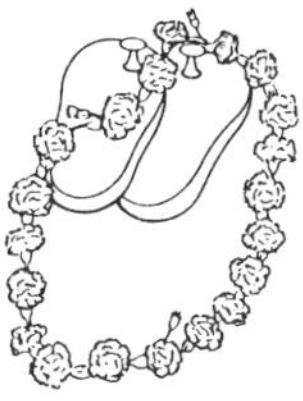

Shri Shri Gurabe Namah
Ohm

Contents

Shri Shri Gurabe Namah
Ohm

Chapter One

Sākṣī (Manifestation)

Jaget Jānāyo yohi sakal, so Guru pragaṭe āye
Yinh āñkhiyanh Guru dekhioñ, so Guru dehiñ lakhāye. ***1.***

It was through the prowess of the Guru (Ātmā, Brahman) that I had so long experienced the transitory (restless) world. But now the Guru has manifested himself before me (in complete tranquillity). The Guru has revealed to me eyes with which I can see Him.

Note: The Prāṇa-Vāyu, which has so long been restless, has now attained a state of perfect calm through Prāṇāyāma received by the Grace of Shriguru. The mind, therefore, has shaken off its restlessness and is securely seated at the Lotus Feet of the Ātmā. For this Self-Realization it was essential that the Guru should graciously open my spiritual eye (divya drṣṭi: physically, the concentration of gaze in the two-petalled lotus in between the eye-brows) through his divine power. The Guru thus is identical with the Ātmā ('Ātmā vai Gururekah' – the Ātmā or God is the only Guru and ultimately makes the disciple, too, identical with the Ātmā or Saccidānanda).

Kabīr bhali bheñi yo Guru mile, nehito hoti hāni
Dīpak jyoti patang yeño, bartā pûrā jāni. ***2.***

Kabīr says that it is very good that he has got a Guru. Otherwise he would have to lose himself like an insect who throws itself into the flame of a lamp, and dies.

Note: The Guru is one who leads the disciple from the darkness of ignorance and attachment to the light of divine consciousness. As insects are enchanted by the light of the lamp and get lost, so a man without having knowledge of the Ātmā is burnt by the false glare and dazzle of earthly attachment and vain pleasures. It is only through the Grace of the Guru that one understands one's mistake and is saved from bondage.

Kabīr bhali bheñi yo Guru mile, yinhate pāte jāuñ
Ghaṭhi māha cautarā, ghaṭhi māha dewān. **3.**

Kabīr says that it is very fortunate that he has received the contact of Shriguru and obtained wisdom from him. It is the Guru who has shown him the Supreme king (God) on his throne in the vessel of the body.

Note: Man obtains wisdom when he knows the Ātmā. Within the head there is an altar with an illumined throne. 'Dewān' means an officer entrusted with the responsibility of managing an estate. Here it refers to the 'Jīvātmā, the human consciousness, which, when it surrenders before God, can have all this experience.

Kabīr Guru guruā milā baliyāyā ḍhelauon
Jātipāñti kul meṭigei nām dharāoye kaun. **4.**

Kabīr says that the Sadguru has been available. As a clod of earth is turned by force into particles of dust, so through the force of the Sadguru attachment to caste, creed and community is absolutely broken. Who, then, will be able to lead us any more to the tie of names (i.e., names and shapes, or the world of objective reality)?

Note: When due to the Grace of Shriguru the Jīvātmā is united with the Paramātmā, everything turns out to be the Brahman or Paramātmā. This is what is called "Kriyār para avasthā" (the stage after the Kriyās, i.e. when all the Kriyās or processes of Yoga have been practiced and one has attained to a state of consciousness transcending the Kriyās) by Yogiraj Shri Shri Shyama Charan Lahiri Mahashay. At that stage nothing in the so-called objective world has its separate name, shape or properties, but everything is merged in one all-embracing Divine consciousness. Spiritually, there is nothing existent but God. It is He who is everything and everywhere.

Kabīr jñān prakāśī Guru mile so Guru bisri nā yāy
Yab Govind dayā kari, tab Guru mili yāy. **5.**

Kabīr says that the Guru who reveals the Supreme Knowledge can never be forgotten. It is only through Divine Grace that a contact with Sadguru can be established.

Note: The Ātmā can be realized within this body at the transcendent stage ('Kriyār para avasthā') which can only be achieved through the Grace of the Guru.

Kabīr Guru Govind dvau ek hāy, dujā hāy ākār
Āpāñ mete Hari bhajei, tab pāoye kartār. **6.**

Kabīr says that the Guru and Govinda (the Divine) are actually one, although they have different shapes. When the ego subsides, one worships Hari (the Lord) and reaches Him.

Note: The Jīvātmā and the Paramātmā are the Kriyā and the state of consciousness after the Kriyā. They are different stages of the same Reality. It is through the Kriyā (Jīvātmā) that one receives the Transcendent consciousness or the Paramātmā.

Kabīr Guru Govind dvau khāṛe. kāke lagoñ pāy
Balihāri Guru Āpne, yinha Govind diyā lakhāy. *7.*

"If the Guru and Govinda are both present, 'Who', asks Kabīr, 'is to be saluted first?'" Kabīr says that the Guru is to be worshipped first, for it is he who has shown Govinda.

Note: It is Jīvātmā who is to be worshipped first. Long practices of Kriyā lead us to the Ājñā Cakra or *Kûṭastha.

It is then that we realize the Jīvātmā. Prolonged meditation in the Kûṭastha again leads us gradually to Sahasrāra (the thousand-petalled Lotus within the head) which is the special seat of the Paramātmā within the body. The word Guru is often used as identical with the Paramātmā. But it may also be used in the sense of Jīvātmā, or, in the physical world, the Master who shows us the path of the Paramātmā. When one reaches the Paramātmā or the

---

***Kûtasṭha actually means the anvil of the blacksmith. It is on the anvil that the blacksmith gives shapes to different things. But the anvil itself remains unchanged. So also is the Divine who is the only unchangeable Reality, while everything in the Universe is in a constant state of flux. The word Kûtasṭha, however, can refer both to Jīvātmā and Paramātmā.**

Transcendent consciousness, there is no more any necessity for the Kriyās. But just because it is the Kriyās which ultimately lead us to a stage transcending the Kriyās, therefore, they are of primary importance.

Kabīr balihāri Guru Āpne, ghaṛi ghaṛi śawār
Mānukhteñ devtā kiyo karat nā lāgi bār. ***8.***

Kabīr thanks his Guru a thousand times, for it is he who can make man a god every moment and a hundred thousand times. He does not take time to do it.

Note: The Kriyā given by the Guru leads us every moment nearer to perfection.

Kabīr sanśay khāyā sakal jag, sanśay koi nā khāy
Yo bedhā Guru acchar, so sanśay cuni khāy. ***9.***

Kabīr says that doubt has devoured up the whole world, but nobody has devoured doubt. One who has understood the true nature of the Guru and the Akṣara Brahman (the Unchangeable Reality, the Paramātmā) has actually eaten up doubt completely.

Note: When, after a long practice of Kriyā, a man reaches the state of perfect tranquillity, doubt is totally dispelled, and the realization dawns upon him that he himself is in everything and everything is within himself. He realizes the identity of the Guru and God.

Kabīr buṛethe pheri ubre, Guru ki lahari camki
Berā dekhā jhāñjherā, utrike bhaye pharki. ***10.***

Kabīr says that he had got already drowned, but a wave made by the Guru saved him from death. He saw a boat full of innumerable holes, and therefore, in fear, he kept aloof from it.

Note: Man remains drowned in the Ocean of ignorance or Māyā. It is the Guru who holds him up. Then he realizes that anything in this physical world is like a boat with countless holes in it and is therefore thoroughly undependable.

Kabīr ek nāmke paṭtare devekoñ kuch nāhi
Kyāle Guruhi samdhiye, hāus rahe man māhi. ***11.***

Kabīr says that such a name (state) has arisen that the disciple has nothing to offer to his Shriguru. They have been completely identified. Unless there are two, how can one offer something to the other? The desire for addressing the Guru is, therefore, not fulfilled.

Note: When the Jīvātmā is identified with the Paramātmā, there is but one Name (i.e., the Paramātmā). This happens at the state of transcending the Kriyās. The false 'I' is eliminated and it is only the alter-ego that remains.

Kabīr man diyā tinhuñ sab diyā, manke sāth śarīr
Āb devekoñ kyā rahā, eoñ kahe dās Kabīr. ***12.***

Kabīr says that he has surrendered both his mind and body. He has given his all. What else could be given?

Note: When, after a long practice of Kriyās, the devotee transcends his limited self and merges it in an unlimited Consciousness, it may be said that he has given himself totally over to the Paramātmā. It is this transcendent stage which is called 'Kriyār para avasthā' where there is no separate existence of the devotee from the points of view of Consciousness and Bliss.

Kabīr śikligar kījiye śabda, maskalā dei
Mankā mayil choṛāike, citdarpaṇ karilei. ***13.***

('Śikligar' means cleansing the weapons).

Kabīr says: "Cleanse the weapons. At the time of washing and cleansing the weapons a sound is heard. But after the weapons are made clean, there is no such sound. The mind also should be cleansed likewise in order to make it like a mirror."

Note: When somebody removes the rust from a weapon, what he does is to repeat his cleansing process from the tip of the weapon to its tail, and back again from the tail to the tip. A sound also is emitted at this time. So also when the mind is cleansed by Paramātmā, what the Sādhaka does is to move his Prāṇa-Vāyu from Mūlādhāra to Sahasrāra and again from Sahasrāra to Mūlādhāra, and the sound of Prāṇāyāma is heard in the process. But when the mind gets tranquil and merged in the Paramātmā, there is no restlessness, and the mind at such a stage serves the purpose of a mirror on which the reflection of the Divine rests spontaneously and with ease.

Kabīr Guru dhobi, śikh kāpṛā, sāban srjni hār
Surtī śilāpar dhoie, nikle jyoti apār. ***14.***

Kabīr says that the Guru is like the washerman and the disciple the clothes to be washed. The Supreme Lord and Creator is the soap and meditation of the Divine is the slab of stone on which the clothes are washed. The disciple, thus washed with Divine consciousness, becomes clean and blessed with Divine light.

Note: The Guru cleanses the mind of the disciple with Kriyā, by charging him with Divine energy. When through repeated practices of Kriyā, the earthly attachments of the mind gradually wear off, the disciple feels the Blessed Light of Paramātmā within himself.

Kabīr ghar baiṭhe Guru pāyā, baṛe hāmāre bhāg
Soi ko tarsat hate, āb amarat āñcāon lāg. ***15.***

Kabīr says that he is highly fortunate in having the Guru near at hand. There was a time when even with great efforts he could not procure the most insignificant thing, but now he has Divine Bliss, enough and to spare.

Note: Kabīr says that the Ātmā is our Guru, and we can realize Him in our own bodies. After Self-Realization one can initiate others too in Kriyā which finally leads to the same Realization.

Kabīr guruko lāl gaṛāoñ kare, matin pakaṛai heta
Ek khoñṭ lāgā rahe, yao lagi lahe nā bhed. ***16.***

Kabīr says that if there would be no impediment of dust (i.e., the body), he would transform the body into 'lāl' (a valuable stone, i.e., something permanent). So long as this difficulty remains, it is essential that we should stick to One (viz., Paramātmā).

Note: Even when one reaches the Paramātmā, the human body remains human in the shape of flesh and blood. But in the spiritual sense even the body, though physical, is really identified with the Ātmā, and illumined with divine consciousness.

Kabīr Guru ko lāl śikhku bhañi, gaṛi gaṛi kāṛe khot
Antar hate sāhār dei, bāher bāher coṭ. ***17.***

Kabīr says: "The Guru always remains 'lāl' or valuable, but the disciple is every moment being engaged in fruitless controversies, i.e., evil propensities. The disciple reacts at every sense-impression received from the outside world."

Note: The Ātmā always remains non-attached, changeless through all circumstances. It is the mind which, although it touches the transcendent state or the Ātmā sometimes, has always the tendency to come down and be involved in earthly attachment. Here the Guru stands for the Ātmā and the disciple for the mind. It is only after a long practice that the mind, through divine Grace, reaches the Brahman. Before that, the mind has its alternate rises and falls to and from the state of absolute tranquillity or 'Kriyār para avasthā'.

Kabīr Jñān samāgam premasukh, dayā bhakti biśwās
Guru sevāte pāyie, satguru śabda nevās. ***18.***

Kabīr says that experience of the divine comes to a man who has mercy, devotion and faith. Such experience leads him to the Bliss of Divine Love. Faithful service to Shriguru elicits instructions from him and when one follows those instructions without hesitation, one experiences Divine Bliss.

Note: The experience of the purely tranquil state is tasting Divine Love. When somebody, after experiencing this Love, tries to make others taste this also, he is said to have mercy. Having this mercy he finds that other people too are attaining the same happiness. This increases his devotion and gradually he attains Supreme Faith in the Eternal Reality. All this can only be attained by being a follower of the Ātmā through Kriyās.

Kabīr Guru mānukh kari jānte, te nar kahiye andh
Ihañ duhkhī samsār me, āge Yamko bānd. ***19.***

Kabīr says that one who thinks of the Sadguru as a human being is a blind fellow. He is unhappy in this life and will be tied by Yama (the god of death) in the life hereafter, i.e., he will be a slave to the cycle of birth and death.

Note: The Sadguru is unified with the Divine and therefore should never be taken as a mere human being. It is only by following the instructions (the Kriyā, the Sādhanā) of such a God-man that one can have liberation from the bondage of worldly attachment.

Kabīr Guru mānukh kari jānte, carṇāmrta ko pān
Te nar narak hi Yāhenge, janma janma hoye śoyān. ***20.***

Kabīr says that a man who drinks the feet-wash of the Guru thinking of him as a mere human being will go to hell and will be born again and again as a dog.

Note: The water which has washed the Feet of the Sadguru is considered to be holy and is taken by the disciple with utter devotion. The statement has a deeper spiritual meaning underneath, although even physically taking such water has great spiritual effects. The nectar of the Feet of Shriguru spiritually implies the nectar that oozes from the Sahasrāra, the special seat of the Ātmā or Brahman within the head. This nectar can only be tasted by one who has reached the transcendent stage after a long practice of the Kriyās. Unless this is attained, complete liberation from animality cannot be obtained.

Kabīr te nar adha hāy, Guru koñ kahate āor
Hari ruṭhe Guru smaran hāy, Guru ruṭhe nahi ṭhaor. ***21.***

Kabīr says that one who takes the Guru as different from the Paramātmā is a low sort of a man. If Hari (God) is displeased, the Guru can still save the disciple by pleasing the Divine, but if the Guru himself is displeased, there remains no shelter for the disciple.

Note: If the devotee falls down from the perfectly tranquil state, he can regain it if he sticks to his practice of the Kriyās. But if he abandons Kriyā itself, there is no hope of his ever attaining the transcendent state ('Kriyār para avasthā').

Kabīr Guru mātheteñ utre, śabda bihunā hoy
Tāko Kāl Ghaseti hai, rākhi śake nāhi koy. **22.**

Kabīr says that if the Guru descends from the head, the Divine Absorption is broken and thus the Anāhata sound is stopped. In that case Time will drag the devotee down and nobody can save him.

Note: When Kriyā is stopped, the mind can no more reach the Sahasrāra, and gradually it is led astray by worldly attachments.

Kabīr aham agni hrday dahe, Gurute cāhe mān
Tinhako Yam neotā diyā, tom houhu mere mejmān. **23.**

Kabīr says that when the fire of egotism burns the heart, the disciple craves for honor even from Shriguru. Such a person, however, becomes a favorite to Yama, the god of death. (That is, he is on the surest path of destruction).

Note: One who has no concentration on the Kûṭastha is assailed by pride and egoism. But his pride deviates him from the path of the Divine and thus leads to his downfall.

Kabīr Guru pāraś Guru pāraś, hay, Guru candan subās
Sat Guru pāraś jīuke, yinho dinho mukti newās. **24.**

Kabīr says that the Guru is the touchstone and he is the fragrant sandalwood. Sadguru is the touchstone for man, for it is he who gives man the shelter for liberation.

Note: The touchstone turns base metals into gold. So also the Guru transforms the disciple. Just because the Guru is constantly in the Brahman, the Divine Fragrance is always with him and so he is compared to the sandalwood. It is the Guru who leads the disciple into the transcendent state of consciousness (Kriyār para avasthā), the state of complete liberation from all kinds of bondage.

Kabīr Guru pāraś me bhed hāy, baro antaro jān
Yohañ loha Kāncan kare, ye e Kañrilei āpu Samān. **25.**

Kabīr says that there is great difference between a touchstone and the Guru, for a touchstone transforms iron only into gold, but the Sadguru makes the disciple his own equal.

Note: The Guru is infinitely superior to the touchstone, because he raises his disciple to the highest level of consciousness, where the Guru and the disciple get identified.

Kabīr Guruko kijiye danḍavat, koṭi koṭi parṇām
Jyā ese bhrngī kīt ko, karle āpu samān. ***26.***

Kabīr wants to offer innumerable pranāms to the Guru. As the goldworm transforms the cockroach into another goldworm, so the Guru transforms the disciple into his own second self.

Note: If the disciple practices the Kriyā and concentrates on the Ājñā Cakra (the point in between the eye-brows) or the Kûṭastha, he, through the grace of Shriguru, gradually reaches the Paramātmā and becomes the Guru himself.

Kabīr Guruko tan man dijiye, mukti padārath jāni
Guru ki sevā mukti phal, yeha Girihī sahi dānī. ***27.***

Kabīr says that the body and mind should be totally surrendered to Shriguru. That is liberation. And the result of liberation again is rendering service to the Guru. Whether a householder or a giver of riches, service to Shriguru is everything.

Note: Kriyā is the process of surrendering body and soul to Shriguru or Paramātmā. And once the surrender is complete, i.e., once the devotee reaches "Kriyār para avasthā", there is liberation for him from bondage.

Kabīr Guru soñ bhed yo lijiye, śis dijiye dān
Bahutak avadhū bahi gyāye, rākhe jīu abhimān. ***28.***

Kabīr says that only the disciple who has already given his head to the Guru (i.e., has already made a complete surrender to the Master's will) can have the deepest spiritual knowledge. Many avadhūtas (Sannyāsins) have been washed away by the strong current of the Ocean of earthly existence only because they could not surrender their ego.

Note: The Prāṇa-Vāyu settles within the head at the transcendent stage (Kriyār para avasthā). That is the state of total surrender to Shriguru or of complete identification with him.

Kabīr Guruko sarvasva dijiye, aor puchiye arthāe.
Kahe Kabīr pad par soi, so hamsā ghare yāe. ***29.***

Kabīr says that in order to attain the Knowledge of the Self a man has to surrender his all to the Guru. Such a devotee touches the Feet of the Infinite and enters the region of the Swan (i.e., the special seat of the Brahman within the head).

Note: When through the practice of Kriyās the devotee feels the presence of the Ātmā everywhere, only then can it be said about him that he has surrendered his all to the Divine. In such a state of consciousness he enters the Sahasrāra, the seat of the Hamsa (Paramātmā) and gets identified with him. 'Hamsa' symbolizes the intake (ham) and outpour (sah) of breath or Prāṇa-Vāyu and Brahman is the prime source of this process. It is also taken as the opposite of "सोऽहम्" (Soham) or " I am He". In the highest state the human consciousness is merged with the Divine consciousness and therefore both "He is I" and "I am He" are correct from the point of view of the devotee. The word "Hamsa" also means the 'swan'. Just as the swan roams about on the surface of water and is yet not merged in it, so also the Paramātmā is within our body, and yet he is not attached to it.

Kabīr Guru gamya batāoye nehi śikh gahe nehiñ khuṭ
Lok bhed bhākhe nehiñ, so Guru Kāyer ṭhunṭ. ***30.***

Kabīr says that a Guru who cannot show his disciple the proper path or reveal before him the prop along which he will have to proceed to the Divine, is a useless as a man without hands.

Note: It is the Guru who teaches the disciple to canalize his Prāṇa-Vāyu through the Suṣumnā, the delicate passage through the spinal cord. The spine may be described as the prop or the pillar along which the disciple would proceed to the Sahasrāra where actually he will attain to perfect tranquillity and bliss.

Kabīr Guru batāyeñ sādhuko, sādhu kahe Guru bujh
Āraś paraśke madhime, bhai āgam ki sujh. ***31.***

Kabīr says that the Guru (Ātmā) instructs the Sādhu (Saint, the Guru in the human frame) and the Sādhu asks his disciple to understand the real Guru (Ātmā). When the disciple meets his Master and receives his blessed touch, he realizes the true meaning of the Scriptures.

Note: The human Guru is always guided by the Divine. The Guru leads his disciple to "Kriyār para avasthā" or the Transcendent state of consciousness. It is then that the devotee understands the mystery of the Āgama the ('Śāstra's or the Scriptures) and there is a union between the Jīvātmā and the Paramātmā.

Kabīr Guru samān dātā nāhiñ, yācak śikh samān
Tin lokki sampradā, so Guru dinho dān. ***32.***

Kabīr says that there is no giver like the Guru and no receiver like the disciple. The Guru bestows all the wealth belonging to the three worlds (i.e., 'svarga' or heaven, 'martya' or earth, and pātāla or the nether region) upon the disciple.

Note: The Brahman or the Paramātmā is everything in this universe. The Guru, therefore, by showing the way to the Paramātmā (the Divine) gives everything to his disciple. The Kriyā given by the Guru makes the disciple rotate in the three worlds within the body. From the navel to the legs is the region Pātāla, from the navel to the throat is the region of this Earth and from the throat to the Ājñā Cakra is the region of Heaven. The devotee moves in all three worlds through the Prāṇāyāma.

Kabīr pahile dātā śikh bhaye, tan man arpo śis
Pāche dātā Guru bhaye, nām diyā bakhśiś. ***33.***

Kabīr says that it is the disciple who first becomes the bestower, because it is he who offers his body and mind to the Guru. Only then does the Guru grant him the Name of the Divine.

Note: To practice Kriyā is to surrender body and mind to the Divine. It is through the Kriyā that the devotee reaches the Kingdom of heaven within his body and listens to the celestial music which may be described as Anāhata Nāda (the sound not artificially generated) or the Name of the Divine.

Chapter 2

Ascertaining the real Guru

Kabīr guru lobhī śikh lalcī, dono khele dāño
Dono buṛe bāpure caṛi pātthal ki nāoñ. ***1.***

Kabīr says that a greedy guru and an avaricious disciple are both for mean practical gain. In such cases both the guru and the disciple sail as it were in a boat made of stone and get easily drowned.

Note: If the guru and the disciple are both enchanted by earthly desires, their minds and Prāṇa-Vāyu roam about in the nether Cakras (plexuses) in the lower parts of the body and they gradually get involved in sinful activities.

Kabīr yāko guru hāy āñdhrā, cela khaṛā nirandh
Andhe andhe ṭheliā duno kūāñ pavant. ***2.***

Kabīr says that where the guru and the disciple are both blind (to the spiritual reality), they jostle with each other and fall into a well.

Note: Where the guru himself is too much attached to earthly enjoyments, he cannot lead the disciple to the higher Kriyās and spiritual consummation.

Kabīr jānā nehi bujhā nehi, pichna kiyā gaon
Andheke andhā milā, path batāoye kon. ***3.***

Kabīr says that one who knows nothing, understands nothing and does not want to gain knowledge from wise persons, is a blind fellow and gains a guru as blind as himself. Who can lead such a man along the proper path?

Note: Unless the guru himself has attained 'Kriyār para avasthā', he has no right to guide a disciple through the path of Kriyā or spiritual Sādhanā.

Kabīr myāy mūṛo, us guruki yateñ bharam nā yāy
Āpne buṛā dhārme, celā diyā bāhāy. ***4.***

Kabīr says that he himself is ignorant, and the guru he has got is also steeped in illusion. His guru therefore is himself immersed in the current (of earthly attachments) and has been the cause of his disciple's drowning. [Of course, Kabīr does not refer to his Guru or to himself in these lines. He takes himself as a representative of the common man here, the blind disciple guided by a blind guru.]

Note: If the guru himself is no real Guru, if his own consciousness has not yet reached tranquillity, how can he lead the disciple to the higher stages of Kriyā?

Kabīr gurunhu bhed hāy, gurunhu me bhāo
So Guru niśu din badiye, yo śabda batāoye dao. ***5.***

Kabīr says that there are distinctions amongst different gurus and their modes of Sādhanā too may be different. Kabīr asks to take the shelter of a Guru who can lead the disciple to the 'Ohm' sound through Prāṇāyāma.

Note: Kabīr says that the best Guru is one who can show the disciple the process leading to the Divine sound of 'Ohm' which can only come to a man when his Prāṇa-Vāyu (breath) can at ease be settled on the Ājñā-Cakra, the plexus in between the eye-brows. This is the highest state of the Kriyās and after this the disciple reaches the Paramātmā or "Kriyār para avasthā".

Kabīr pūre guru vinā, pūrā śikh nā hoye
Guru lobhī śikh lālcī, tāte jhājhni duni śoye. ***6.***

Kabīr says that unless the guru himself has perfect wisdom, the disciple cannot reach spiritual consummation. If the guru hankers only after material gains, and the disciple happens to be of the same category, both of them remain doubly asleep to the spiritual reality.

Note: Unless the Jīvātmā is completely merged in the Paramātmā, the human mind cannot attain perfect tranquillity.

Attachment to the Paramātmā is the only way to curb the distraction of the mind. And for this Kriyā is absolutely essential.

Kabīr pūra sahaje guṇ kare, guṇe naoyāye cheha
Sāyer pokhe sarbhare, dān na māge meha. ***7.***

Kabīr says that with the help of the 'Sahaja' (natural) Kriyāyoga the Guru lifts the mind of the disciple upwards, while through this process again the Paramātmā comes down as it were to grace the devotee. Thus, when a divine communion is established through Kriyāyoga, the disciple gets merged in the Divine consciousness, and as such does not ask for anything. When the giver (Paramātmā) and the receiver (human consciousness) get identified, who will give and who will receive? Just as rivers coming from different directions are united spontaneously with the Ocean and just as clouds bring showers spontaneously on earth, so also the merging of human consciousness with the Divine is made spontaneous through the Kriyās given by the Guru.

Note: Kriyāyoga has been termed "Sahaja Kriyāyoga" by Yogiraj Shri Shri Shyama Charan Lahiri Mahashay. The word "Sahaja" means 'easy' or 'natural'. Kriyāyoga as taught by the Sadguru has nothing artificial or troublesome in it, and as the disciple proceeds upwards, he gradually gets enamoured of the process and finds it 'easy'. 'Sahaja' literally means that which is born or manifested at the very time of our birth. We are born with our respiration, the intake and outpour of breath, and it does not leave us till our death. Hence the process of Sādhanā which is based on Prāṇāyāma has been described as natural and spontaneous. The Guru teaches the process of canalizing the Prāṇa-Vāyu through the Suṣumnā, the very delicate passage through the spinal cord, and, spontaneously, the disciple moves towards the Ocean of Saccidānanda, The attainment of the highest state of consciousness ('Kriyār para avasthā') may be likened to a refreshing shower from dark clouds. The disciple feels illumined at every fibre of his being.

Kabīr pūra sat Guru nā milā, rāhā adhurā śikh
Svā gaj tīkā parhīkai, ghar ghar mānge bhikh. ***8.***

Kabīr says that lack of contact with a perfect Guru leaves the disciple with a fickle mind. Such a restless mind may be compared with the curved figure of an elephant. The disciple with a restless mind is a beggar begging for alms from door to door, i.e., his mind constantly runs after earthly possessions.

Note: The imperfect Guru cannot train the disciple in the process of canalizing the Prāṇa-Vāyu along the straight path, i.e., the Suṣumnā. In ordinary existence the Prāṇa-Vāyu moves through the passages along the left and right sides of the body (the Īṛā and the Pingalā). Kriyā or Sādhanā seeks to make if flow through the straight path (Suṣumnā) within the spinal cord. And this alone is the path which can lead the devotee to "Kriyār para avasthā" or the state of final perfection.

Kabīr pūra sat Guru nā milā, rāhā adhurā śikh
Niksāthā Haribhajan ko, bajhi gyāye māyā bik. ***9.***

Kabīr says that if Sadguru is not available, the disciple cannot attain tranquillity of mind. The disciple was out to worship Hari (Paramātmā), but he is again steeped in Māyā (illusion).

Note: The word "Hari" literally means One who steals away all our troubles and anxieties. The devotee worships the Lord in order to eliminate sorrows and anxieties from life. But this cannot be done unless the straight path is shown by Shriguru.

Kabīr Guru ki bāhār dehakā, sat Guru cinhā nāhi
Bhau sāgar ko jālme, phiri phiri gotā khāi. ***10.***

Kabīr says that we have taken the body as the Guru and do not know the Sadguru himself. That is the reason why we are caught within the net of worldly illusion and are assailed again and again by doubts.

Note: Actually the Ātmā within us is eternal. But due to lack of practice of the Kriyās we identify ourselves with the body and feel joys and sorrows. Our real being is independent of joys and sorrows. But we can never achieve this Self-Realization unless we perform the Kriyās.

Kabīr yohi gurute bhay nā meṭe, bhrānti man ki nā yāy
Guruto yaysā cāhiye, yo dei Brahma darśāy. ***11.***

Kabīr says that he does not want a guru who cannot dispel fear and illusion. A Guru who can make the disciple realize the Brahman is the One who is needed.

Note: The perfect Guru leads the disciple to the completely fearless state of consciousness, the perfect state of bliss or "Kriyār para avasthā". This state can only be reached through a proper training in the Kriyās.

Kabīr kāṇ phukā Guru haddakā, behaddakā Guru aor
Behaddakā Guru yab mile, tao lahe thikānā ṭhāor. ***12.***

Kabīr says that the guru whose activity ceases after uttering Mantras (sacred words which the disciple ought to go on chanting) in the ears of the disciple, cannot be of much help. When the Guru with unlimited spiritual powers will be available, the devotee will reach Brahman through his guidance.

Note: The perfect Guru compels the disciple to move along the path of Kriyā and thus to reach spiritual consummation.

Kabīr jāne Gurukoñ bujhiyā, pyāyṛā diyā batāy
Caltā caltā tāñhā giyā, yāñhā Niranjan Rāy. ***13.***

Kabīr says that the Guru with his wisdom has shown the proper path. Proceeding along that path we reach the Lord who is above all illusions.

Note: The devotee, after a long practice of Kriyās, reaches the Sahasrāra. It is then that he experiences Transcendent Consciousness which is a state of perfect bliss. This is what is called "Kriyār para avasthā".

Kabīr bandhe ko bandhā milā, chuṭe ko ni upāy
Karu sewā nirbandhaki, palme lei choṛāy. ***14.***

Kabīr says that a guru who himself has not yet been able to shake off the bondage of earthly attachments, can never lead the disciple to liberation. It is the Mukta (liberated) Guru who is to be served, for it is he who has the power to lead the disciple to liberation within a moment.

Note: When the disciple, by following the Sadguru, shakes off his dirt and dross and achieves purity of mind, the real Guru can at once lead his consciousness to the highest state.

Kabīr yākā guru hāy grhī celā grhī hoy
Kik kic ke dhoeñ, dāg nā chuṭe koy. ***15.***

Kabīr says that where the guru himself has earthly attachment, the disciple too inculcates the same attachment. Mere water cannot remove the stain of attachment. (It is only Divine consciousness which can remove sins).

Note: The guru who does not constantly live in the Ātmā cannot lead the disciple to the Divine through the proper Kriyās.

Kabīr guru nām hāy gamyakā, śikh śikhile soy
Binu samghat maryād binu, guru śikh nā hoy. ***16.***

Kabīr says that the guru who does not know his destination is a guru by name alone. The Guru must be Ātmārāma (i.e., one whose only joy is in union with the Ātmā or the Divine). It is only then that he can lead the restless mind of the disciple to the highest state of concentration.

Note: The Ātmārāma Guru imparts Kriyā which gradually leads the mind of the disciple from restlessness to tranquillity. Such tranquillity can only be obtained by One's contact with the Paramātmā.

Kabīr Guru āto saste bhaye, Kauṛike, rapcāś
Āpne tanki śudh nāhi, śikh karan ki Āś. ***17.***

Kabīr says that the so-called guru is so cheap that fifty such people can be available at a paltry sum. It is ridiculous to initiate others when one's own body has not been purified.

Note: Fake gurus are always there in a far greater number than real Ones.

Kabīr yo niham acchar pāiya, tākā meṭikā doy
So Guru pūra kahiye, kadihi grhī nā hoy. ***18.***

Kabīr says that the proper Guru reaches the Akṣara (One who has no change or destruction) or Eternal after completely surrendering his own ego. At the highest state of consciousness, therefore, there are no two (The Divine and the human), but One (the Paramātmā). The Guru who has been identified with this Eternal One is the perfect Guru. He may be a family-man, and yet he is a Sannyāsin.

Note: When through the Kriyā we reach even a higher state than the Ājñā Cakra, we reach the Illimitable Zone of One (i.e., the Sahasrāra) and feel the Ātmā or Brahman everywhere. This is 'Kriyār para avasthā', and even if a householder reaches this stage, he remains no householder in the restricted sense, because his home is everywhere since everything is Brahman in his consciousness – "सर्वं खल्विदं ब्रह्म" ।

Kabīr jhuñṭe guru ki pacchukoñ, tyajat na kije bār
Dawār nā pāyoe śabdakā, bharme bhao jaladhār. ***19.***

Kabīr says that one should not delay in abandoning a false guru, beacause such a guru can never lead him to the door of Ohmkāra, the Anāhata Nāda (the sound that is not generated by striking one thing against another: Divine sound) which leads us ultimately to God. In that case the disciple will have to remain steeped in the Ocean of earthly attachment and ignorance.

Note: According to Yogis the human body has six main Cakras, (lotuses or plexuses) within the Suṣumnā: Mūlādhāra just above the anus, Svādhisṭhāna behind the penis, Manipūra at the back of the navel, Anāhata just behind the breast, Viśuddha on the back side of the throat, and Ājñā within the forehead in between the eye-brows. As the Prāṇa-Vāyu settles in each Cakra, particular sounds are heard in each place. It is these sounds which are called the 'Anāhata Nāda's. There may actually be innumerable kinds of such inner sounds, but all these lead gradually to the Ohmkāra (the Ohm sound) which is taken as a compendium of all sounds. It is only when the devotee's mind settles in the Ājñā Cakra that the

Ohmkāra can be heard within. If this sound is heard for a long time, the devotee attains Samādhi (complete absorption in the Divine) and reaches the soundless region within the head which is called Sahasrāra or the thousand-petalled lotus, the special seat of the Lord within the human body. The inner sound "Ohm" therefore is the first manifestation of the Lord in terms of word or sound. As the Bible says, "And in the beginning there was the word and the word was God." The word Ājñā literally means 'order', 'command'. In spiritual Sādhanā it is only when the Ājñā Cakra gives the command, that the human consciousness reaches its consummation and gets identified with the Divine. Thus the Ājñā Cakra may very well be described as the "gateway of the inner world". And the real Guru teaches his disciple the process of concentrating in the Ājñā Cakra.

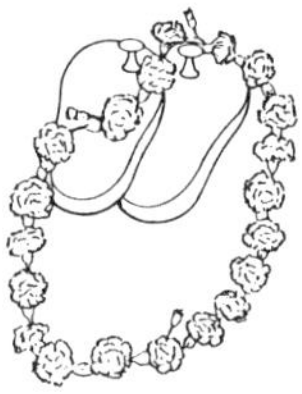

Chapter 3

The Glory of the Sadguru

Kabīr Sat Guru sam kai sang nehi, sādhu sam nāhi jāti
Hari samāne nāhi hita kai, Hari jana sam nāhi pāñti. ***1.***

Kabīr says that there is no company like that of a Sadguru, no class or caste like that of a Sādhu (Saint) no benefactor like Shri Hari (the Lord) and no community like that of persons who always live in Shri Hari (i.e., in God-consciousness).

Note: The Kriyā leads us to the Paramātmā. The Sadguru, identified in consciousness with the Lord, imparts Kriyā to the disciple. That is the greatest gift and therefore contact with the Sadguru is the most blessed contact which leads us ultimately to Peace, Tranquillity and Divine Rapture.

Kabīr Sadguruki mahimā anant hāy, anant kiyā upakār
Locana ananta, udhāria dekhaba nehār. ***2.***

Kabīr says that the Glory of the Sadguru is Illimitable and Indescribable. People receive unlimited benefits from him. The Sadguru's insight and power of vision too is unlimited, and with this vision he makes his disciple experience Brahman within a short time and thus leads him to Liberation from bondage.

Note: The Sadguru who has realized the Ātmā becomes as all-pervasive in his consciousness as the Ātmā Himself and can reveal the Kûṭastha, the Jñāna-netra (eye of knowledge) in his Ājñā-Cakra which enables him to see Divine Effulgence and leads him to the Illimitable in the Sahasrāra.

Kabīr sab jag bharmat ioñ phire, yayoñ jangalka rojh
Sadguru se śodhi bhei, pāyā Harikā khoñj. ***3.***

Kabīr says that the whole world is moving about in ignorance like the man who does not know the herbs (for curing diseases) and yet goes on searching for them in the forest. It is only when the Sadguru will rectify the errors that men will reach the Lord.

Note: It is the Kriyā which purifies the body and the mind and leads the devotee gradually to "Kriyār para avasthā".

Kabīr āti pāi thir bhayo, Sadguru dinhā dhir
Māṇik hīra baṇijiā, mān sarovar tīr. ***4.***

Kabīr says that it is through the Grace of Sadguru that he has reached the state of tranquillity. Trading in jewels and diamonds he has reached the shore of the Mānasa Lake (one of the biggest lakes in the Himalayas, charged with holy associations).

Note: The Sadguru leads the disciple to "Kriyār para avasthā". By practicing Kriyā the devotee reaches the Kûṭastha in the Ājñā Cakra where he experiences 'Jyotih' or Divine Light of variegated colors. This Light Divine has been described as jewels. And the Supreme Lord has been described as a diamond. The Lord is seen at first as the black spot (Kṛṣṇa) in the middle of the Kûṭastha. If the disciple thus concentrates his mind in the Kûṭastha, he reaches the extermity of the lake of Manas (Mind), i.e., his mind gets to its extreme point and merges itself in the Ocean of Saccidānanda.

Kabīr thita pāi man thir bhayā, Sadguru kari sahāy
Ananta kathā jīo ucarai, hidayā ramitā rāy. ***5.***

Kabīr says that the restless mind has become tranquil only through the Grace of the Sadguru and now the devotee is gifted with unlimited expression, for he has found the Lord who resides in the heart.

Note: The Jīva (human being) becomes Śiva (the Lord) through the practice of Kriyās, and the limited expands itself into the unlimited.

Kabīr cetan cauukī baithī kai, Sat Guru dinahu dhīr
Nirbhay hoye nihśanka bhajo, kebal kahe Kabīr. ***6.***

Kabīr says: "Firmly enthroned in Divine Consciousness, practice fearlessly what the sage Sadguru has given you. Practice Kebala Kumbhaka".

Note: The Prāṇāyāma consists of three parts: the Pūraka or intake of breath, the Recaka or outpour of breath and the Kumbhaka or the moment of rest in between Pūraka and Recaka. It is this moment of rest which has to be prolonged through Kriyāyoga, and the period of Kumbhaka is the only period of rest from all sorts of physical and mental activities, from all desires. 'Kebala' means 'alone', 'above all limitations of time, space or quality'. The term refers to the Paramātmā, the Transcendent Reality. The special kind of Prāṇāyāma ('antarmukh' i.e., in which the breath is let out inside the Suṣumnā) practiced in Kriyāyoga is kebala Prāṇāyāma, because it leads man to the Paramātmā in the "Kriyār para avasthā". The Kumbhaka in this Prāṇāyāma is Kebala Kumbhaka.

Kabīr bahe bāhāne yātthe, loka veda ki sāth
Bic hi Sat Guru mili gyāye, dīpak dinho hāth. ***7.***

Kabīr says that he was flowing along the stream of social customs and scriptures. At this time the Sadguru came and gave him a lamp (of knowledge).

Note: The Sadguru, by opening up the Suṣumnā, provides the disciple with the lamp of spiritual consciousness. The disciple then gradually overcomes the narrowness and limitations imposed by customs and traditions. He gets deeper into the mysteries of the Scriptures and stops being guided by their superficial implications.

Kabīr dīpak dinhā labhabi, bātī dai aghaṭ
Pūra ki āoye sāha nā, bahurinā ceri ahaṭ. ***8.***

Kabīr says that the Guru has given the lamp, but it is only when the Paramātmā has added the wick unto it that the disciple sees the full Divine Effulgence. After that he sees nothing inspite of his best attempts.

Note: It is only after a long practice of the Kriyā given by the Guru that the disciple gains the blessed contact with the Paramātmā. Then he is merged completely in the Ocean of Divine

Light in the "Kriyār para avasthā". As this is the highest state of consciousness, there can be nothing beyond this.

Kabīr Sadguru nidhi milāiyā, Sadguru sāhu sudhīr
Nip Yeme sājhi ghane, bāñṭan hār Kabīr. ***9.***

Kabīr says that the Sadguru is the wisest giver, for it is he who has given the best treasure (viz., the Lord). Now Kabīr shares this treasure with his partners.

Note: It is the Sadguru who shows the Kûṭastha to the disciple. The disciple, after reaching perfection, leads others to the path of Sādhanā (spiritual practices).

Kabīr sat hāñm so rijhikei, ek kahā parsang
Bādar bariṣā premkā, bhiji geyā sab ang. ***10.***

Kabīr says that the Sadguru has satisfied the disciple and led him on to a new contact. The disciple has developed such a love for this new company that all his limbs are thoroughly drenched with the shower of love.

Note: The Sadguru, through the Kriyā, leads the disciple to the Lord. The disciple, by constantly living in God-consciousness, receives the highest gratification and becomes identified with God.

Kabīr caupar māri cauhaṭe, sāri kiyā śarīr
Sadguru dāño bātāiye, khele dās Kabīr ***11.***

Kabīr says that he is playing dice by throwing it all around the body. It is the Sadguru who is instructing him to cast his dice and he merely obeys.

Note: The Guru instructs the Ohmkāra Kriyā (the highest Kriyā) in which the Prāṇa-Vāyu moves throughout the body. It is through this that the disciple reaches "Kriyār para avasthā". (The Ohmkāra Kriyā should only be known personally from a Master Yogī).

Kabīr Sadguruke Sadke Kiyā dil āpnekā sāc
Kal yug hāñmse laṛi paṛā, mohakma merā bāc. ***12.***

Kabīr says that the Sadguru does good to the disciple if the latter surrenders himself heart and soul to him. But Kali Yuga (the age of sin) intervenes and tries to develop the hankering after material possessions.

Note: It is through the Kriyā that we reach "Kriyār para avasthā". But for this we have constantly to struggle against sins. The word 'Kali' here stands for sin. The sages divide the evolution of human consciousness into four ages: Satya, Tretā, Dvāpara and Kali. 'Satya' is the age in which human consciousness reaches the utmost perfection. These ages proceed in a cyclic order, from Satya to Kali, and again from Kali to Satya. Kali Yuga is a dark age for human consciousness. Here, however, the word does not refer to the age, but to the darkness and impurity in every human mind.

Kabīr Sadguru sācā surīyā, śabda yo bāhā ek
Lāgāt hi bhayi meṭi geyi, parā kaleje chek. ***13.***

Kabīr says that the Sadguru is the real Divine tune, for it is he who tunes the life of the disciple to the note of Ohmkāra. And when Ohmkāra is attained, the Prāṇa is no more restless.

Note: When the devotee listens constantly to the sound of Ohmkāra, he attains Samādhi and becomes completely fearless.

Kabīr Sadguru Śabda kamān leli, bāñhan lāge tīr
Ek yo bāhā prīti kari, bedhā sakal śarīr. ***14.***

Kabīr says that the Guru taught the process of shooting arrows (Prāṇāyāma and other Kriyās) with the help of the bow of Ohmkāra. Once the arrows are shot with devotion, the entire body is pierced.

Note: Prāṇāyāma circulates Prāṇa-Vāyu throughout the body. This leads gradually to 'Kriyār para avasthā'.

Kabīr Sadguru mārā bāṇ bharl, dhari kai sudhī muṭhi
Anga ughāre lāgiā, gayā dubhāṣā phuṭi. ***15.***

Kabīr says that the Sadguru taught the process of piercing the target (Paramātmā) through the Kriyās. Once the target is reached, all sense of duality is eliminated.

Note: When the Prāṇa-Vāyu reaches the head through the Suṣumnā, the devotee achieves complete identification with the Paramātmā and therefore the distinction between the knower and the knowable, between the worshipper and the worshipped, completely vanishes. This is the transcendent stage of consciousness (Kriyār para avasthā) where the devotee reaches spiritual consummation.

Kabīr hamse na bole unmanī, cacañl mailā mārī
Kahe Kabīr antar bedhā, Sadgurukā bātiāri. ***16.***

Kabīr says that when the 'Unmanī' (a stage where the mind reaches upwards and settles in the Sahasrāra) stage is reached, the disciple does not even like to talk. For him the moving panorama of life does no more have its separate existence, because the Sadguru has pierced everything with his weapon (viz, Kriyā).

Note: Through a long practice of Kriyās diversion of mind is completely eliminated and the consciousness gets merged into the Divine.

Kabīr guñā huā bāurā, bahirā huā kaṇ
Pāothete pangula huā, Sat Guru marā bāṇ. ***17.***

Kabīr says that the Master has flung the arrows with such intensity that he has no desire to talk. He has the power to hear and yet he does not listen to anything; he has legs and yet, like a paralyzed man, he cannot walk.

Note: When the disciple through a long practice of Kriyās reaches Kriyār para avasthā for the first time, almost all his physical movements remain suspended. Of course, after a prolonged and continued stay in the highest stage of consciousness, Saints grow habituated to Samādhi and regain the necessary movements of their limbs.

Kabīr Guru mera śuruāñ,bedhā sakal śarīr
Bāṇ dubhāṣā chuṭi geyā, keño jīye dās Kabīr. ***18.***

Kabīr says that the Guru is a brave hero who has pierced the entire body of the disciple with arrows, and thus dispelled all sense of duality (i.e., the feeling of separation between the Jīvātmā and the Paramātmā) from him. How could Kabīr now lead his individual existence? (He has got identified with the Divine in his consciousness, and therefore has no separate human consciousness.)

Note: Prāṇāyāma leads ultimately to a state of utter tranquillity, a state of absolute oneness which is "Kriyār para avasthā".

Kabīr Sat Guru sāñcā śuriāñ, nakh śikh mārā pūr
Bāhār dhāoyān diśai, bhitar cāknā cūr. ***19.***

Kabīr says that the Sadguru is the real hero, for he has shot the disciple from head to foot. From the outside the devotee seems to be perfectly all right, although he is smashed inwards.

Note: The power of the Sadguru makes the Prāṇa-Vāyu still and this makes the disciple concentrated in the Divine. At this stage the limited ego is completely merged in the Infinite consciousness.

Kabīr Sat Guru mārā bāṇ bhari, ṭuṭi geyi sab jeb
Kahi āśā kahi āpadā, kahi tasbi kahi kiteb. ***20.***

Kabīr says that the Sadguru has shot his arrows which have destroyed everything (i.e., all earthly conflicts and attachments). Before this, the disciple would sometimes be full of hope, sometimes he would get involved in difficulties due to his own actions, sometimes he would mutter sacred names with the help of a rosary, and sometimes he would suffer from doubts arising out of an improper understanding of the Scriptures.

Note: Before practicing Kriyās a man either remains steeped in worldly attachments or even if he has a mind to worship God, he takes recourse to a thousand and one methods for want of a proper guidance. But after his initiation by the proper Guru he goes on practicing Kriyās till at last he reaches "Kriyār para avasthā" when nothing can disturb his tranquillity.

Kabīr Sat Guru mārā jñān kari, śabda surange bāṇ
Mera māyā phiri jīue, to hāth na gahi kāmān. ***21.***

Kabīr says: "The able Master aimed his arrow at the source of Ohmkāra. He thereby killed me (i.e., my ego). But even if I am alive, I shall no more wield the bow."

Note: Prolonged practice of Kriyās leads to annihilation of the ego. Even if it remains in practical life, it is a shadow of the former ego. It is an ego sublimated by total surrender to the Divine and as such can no more lead man to worldly attachment.

Kabīr Sat Guru mārā bāṇ, nirakhi nirakhi nij thāor
Rām akhilme ramj rāhā, cet nahi āoye āor. ***22.***

Kabīr says that the Sadguru throws the arrow, concentrating his gaze on the Ātmā. When the disciple sees the Ātmā everywhere, his mind reaches the Infinite.

Note: When the Prāṇa-Vāyu flows through the channel of the Suṣumnā and becomes steady within the head, the disciple reaches "Kriyār para avasthā". At this stage everything seems to be a manifestation of the Brahman (Ātmā), and the mind can experience nothing else.

Kabīr Sat Guru wāhi prīti kari, rahi kāṭāri ṭuṭi
Yāysi ani nasālai, tyāysi chālai muṭi. ***23.***

Kabīr says that weapon (instrument) which leads to our union with the Paramātmā is broken. The weapon here refers to the Prāṇa-Vāyu and the breaking is that of its normal flow when the breath becomes still. The mind gets concentrated to the extent to which the Prāṇa-Vāyu becomes steady (symbolized by the "folded palm").

Note: It is due to the restlesness of the breath that the human mind constantly moves on from one object to another. As through the practice of Kriyās the movement of breath is regulated, the mind attains to a greater and greater calm till at last it is completely merged in Divine consciousness in the "Kriyār para avasthā".

Kabīr mān baṛāi ūrume, ei jagko byābahār
Das garibi bandgi, Sat Guru ko upakār. ***24.***

Kabīr says that earthly honor, prestige and egotism – these are generally the ways of the world. But modesty, decency and thought for the well-being of everybody – these are the benefits received from the Sadguru.

Note: When the Prāṇa-Vāyu becomes steady at the Kûṭastha, the Sādhaka attains to a state of profound humility, because he feels the presence of the Divine in every human body and therefore shows proper honor to others. He also tries to propagate Kriyāyoga for the welfare of humanity.

Kabīr dil hi māho dīdar hāy, bād bake Samsār
Sat Guru śabda kām sakalā, yise oyār hi pār. ***25.***

Kabīr says that everything is there in the mind itself, and yet people quarrel amongst themselves for triflings. When due to the grace of Sadguru the sound of Ohmkāra is heard, the devotee can realize both sides of a thing and therefore no cause for quarrel exists for him.

Note: The Kriyā leads man ultimately to Brahman where all contradictions are resolved and the devotee attains to a perfect state of tranquillity which has been described as "Kriyār para avasthā" by Yogiraj Shri Shri Shyama Charan Lahiri Mahashay.

Kabīr yo diśe soi binuśe, nām dharā so yāy
Kahe Kabīr soi tattva gaho, yo Sadguru dei batāy. ***26.***

Kabīr says that everything in this visible world is destructible. Anything that can be described must vanish some day. Kabīr therefore advises us to receive initiation in the path of the Divine. Such initiation can only be had from an able Master.

Note: The Divine is the only Eternal Reality which can be realized at "Kriyār para avasthā". For this again, initiation from a Sadguru and a long and sincere practice of Kriyās is essential.

Kabīr kudrat pāyi khabar soñ, Sadguru dayi batāy
Bhaura bilamba kaulme, ab kyāyseñ uṛi yāy. ***27.***

Kabīr says that the disciple knows the whereabouts of the miraculous Divine Power from the Sadguru. The black bee in order to taste the honey of the lotus goes within its petals, gets drunk and is kept confined within the flower when at sunset the lotus closes its petals. So also the human mind, after having the trace of the Divine Force, gets entangled in it and loses its restlessness.

Note: 'Kula-kuṇḍalinī' is the name of the latent Divine Force in the human body. Through practices in Kriyāyoga this latent Force is awakened, and flows through the Suṣumnā. When the mind, through Kriyās, gets in touch with this Force, it becomes concentrated and still.

Kabīr Rām nām chāṛoñ nahi, Sadguru śikh deyi
Abināśī so paraś kari, Ātmā amar bheyi. ***28.***

Kabīr says: "Never leave off the name of Rāma (the Lord) given to you by the Guru. Once you touch the changeless Reality, you too become immortal".

Note: Taking the name of the Lord is not a mere physical process. The real name of God is the sound of Ohmkāra which can only come within through a devoted practice of Kriyās. It is through the Kriyās that the devotee at last reaches 'Kriyār para avasthā' which is immortality in the real sense of the term.

Kabīr cauṣaṭṭi dīyā yo e kari, caudaha candāñ māhi
Tehi ghar kyāysā candāñ, yohi ghar Sadguru nāhi. ***29.***

Kabīr says that due to absence of the proper Guru the room of our body cannot be lighted although we may have as many as 64 lamps and 14 moons.

Note: We can feel the Divine Light when 64 nerves in our body run in eight different directions and when 14 spheres in our body meet at the root of the tongue, i.e., when we practice Kriyās through the Khecarī Mudrā in which the tongue enters the subtle passage just behind the Ājñā Cakra. But the most proper realization of the Sadguru can only be had at the "Kriyār para avasthā which happens when the Prāṇa-Vāyu becomes still within the head. This is the final stage of Self-Realization or God-Realization.

Kabīr koṭi ek candāñ ugahiñ sūraj koṭi hājār
Kahe Kabīr Sadguru binā, diśai ghor āndhār. ***30.***

Kabīr says: "Even if a *crore of moons and a thousand crores of Suns rise together, darkness cannot be dispelled without the Grace of Sadguru."

*** A crore is the sum of ten million.**

Note: Without the Grace of the Master the resplendent Divine Light cannot be seen in the Kûṭastha. The Light Divine, when it manifests itself in full glory to the devotee, has the intensity of thousands of Suns and at the same time the coolness of thousands of moons.

Kabīr Sadguru mohi neoā jīyā, dinhu su amar bol
Śītal chāyā saghan phal, hamsā karhi kalol. ***31.***

Kabīr says that the Sadguru has saved him with his beautiful and immortal sayings. It is due to the Guru that he has gained the ripe friut of a cool shade. Now the Swan is making sweet sounds in this shade.

Note: The Kriyā obtained from Shriguru leads the disciple, through the Anāhata sounds to direct Realization. The experience of the Divine can always be had in the Transcendent stage which again can never be reached without the help of the Kriyās.

Kabīr Sat Guru sat Kabīr hāy, samkat pareñ hujur
Cukā seobā bandegi, kiyā cākrī dūr. ***32.***

Kabīr says that the Sadguru has identified himself with Kabīr, for he has removed all dangers. If you do not serve him (i.e., if you do not practice Kriyās), he will dismiss you from service.

Note: The Guru, by imparting Kriyāyoga, has eliminated all evil. If the disciple does not engage himself in practicing Kriyās, he will be deprived of Joy Divine.

Kabīr cit cokṣe man ujle, dayābanta gambhīr
Sei dhoke bicle nāhi, yehi Sat Guru mileñ Kabīr. ***33.***

Kabīr says that when the mind becomes pure and illumined, the devotee attains kindness and tranquillity. In this state of consciousness he is never upset by anything, because he has been identified with the Sadguru.

Note: The practice of Kriyās leads gradually to "Kriyār para avasthā" when the devotee reaches a state of complete calm and purity.

Kabīr jñān Samāgam prema sukh, dayā bhakti biśwas
Satguru mili ek bhayā, rahi na duji āś. ***34.***

Kabīr says that when Wisdom comes, the disciple tastes the Joy of Love Divine and attains kindness, devotion and Faith. Because of his identification with the Master he abandons all earthly hope.

Note: With the attaining of the knowledge of Brahman, everything becomes full of Joy. When the realization that everything is Brahman dawns upon the devotee, he gets identified with the Divine and therefore cannot hanker after anything.

Kabīr Sat Guru pāraśko śila, dekha tattva vicāri
Ahi parośini le cali, diyā diyā so bāri. ***35.***

Kabīr says that if you analyze the truth, you will understand that the Sadguru is the real touchstone. As one lamp lights another, so the holy touch of Shriguru lights the divine light in other men.

Note: It is the Sadguru who lights up the Divine consciousness latent in man, by imparting Kriyā.

Kabīr Sat Guru gami yo kahi diyā bhed diyā ār thāy
Surati kaoyalke antaric, nirādhar pad pāy. ***36.***

Kabīr says that the Master has imparted his instruction only after he has had his own realization. He now leads his disciple to the thousand-petalled lotus (Sahasrāra) within the head where he gets identified with the Illimitable.

Note: In the "Kriyār para avasthā", the Prāṇa-Vāyu reaches the head and settles there. This, however, can only be attained through the Grace of the Guru and through a long practice of the Kriyās imparted by the Guru himself.

Kabīr jīv akṣam bahu kuṭil hāy, koi nahi gati āiye
Tāko aygun meṭi kāy, Sat Guru hamsa banāye. ***37.***

Kabīr says that man has no power of his own and his intelligence moves in a round-about manner. He, therefore, knows nothing in its real nature. The Sadguru rectifies all his faults and makes him a real Saint.

Note: Man has really no power. But he realizes his own powerlessness only through his contact with the Divine. And it is the Guru again who makes him establish this contact.

Kabīr Sat Guru baṛe sarāk hāy, parakhe kharāo khoṭ
Bhao sāgarte kāṛike, rākhe āpne Oṭ. ***38.***

Kabīr says that the Sadguru is a great Judge who analyzes the merits and defects of the disciple, snatches him away from the ocean of earthly attachment and takes him within his own fold.

Note: The Guru tests his disciple, and if the latter follows the path shown by the Master with whole-hearted devotion, he reaches the Transcendent state of consciousness.

Kabīr Sat Guru śabda jāhāj hāy, kai kai pāoye bhed
Samudra bund ekai bhayā, kāko karo nikhed. ***39.***

According to Kabīr the Sadguru is like a ship of Ohmkāra. Some people realize it sometimes. When the Ocean and the drop of water become one, who will prevent whom (from getting identified)?

Note: It is through the Kriyās that the sound of Ohmkāra comes within, and gradually, the human consciousness (like a drop of water) reaches complete God-consciousness (like the Ocean) and gets merged into it. The devotee at this stage is left with no fragmentary individual consciousness to be ruffled with earthly joys and sorrows.

Kabīr Sadguru mahal banāīyā, jñān gilāoyā dinha
Dū rī dekhan ke kāraṇe śabd jharokā kinha. ***40.***

Kabīr says that the Sadguru has built a special zone and made his disciple swallow wisdom. He has also purchased a window for listening to Ohmkāra and for seeing things even from a great distance.

Note: The head is the special seat for the Paramātmā within the human body. When, through the Kriyās, the Prāṇa-Vāyu reaches the head, unearthly sights and sounds are experienced by the devotee.

Kabīr Sat Guru vacan māne nāhi, āpni samjhe nāhi
Kahe Kabīr kyā kijiye, kio bithā jio māhi. ***41.***

Kabīr says that a man who himself understands nothing and yet does not follow the instructions of the Sadguru is merely spending a useless human existence.

Note: Human life is superior to all other kinds of life on earth, because it affords the opportunity for Self-Realization. If, therefore, man does not strive after leading a spiritual life, he is no better than a lower animal.

Kabīr Sadguru bāpurā kyā kare, yo śikh hi mohāy cuk
Koṭi yatan pramodhiye, bāñś bājāoye phuk. ***42.***

What, according to Kabīr, can the Master do, if the disciple refuses to be molded? The bamboo, with holes, can only serve as a flute and nothing else.

Note: The will of the disciple to be molded by the Master is as necessary as the Grace of the Guru. The idle disciple merely takes in and lets out breath. He cannot reach the consummation of human existence.

Kabīr Sat Guru milā to kyā bhayā, yo man parlā bhol
Pāś vīṇā ḍhāñkā paṛā, kyā kare bāpurā col. ***43.***

Kabīr says: "Even if Sadguru is available, what can he do for a man who has no mind to serve God? The lyre is just beside him; only it is covered with cloth. If the disciple does not remove the covering cloth and play on the instrument, is it after all the fault of the covering cloth?"

Note: The disciple, too, on his part, must put in his own effort in order to achieve Self-Realization. The Guru might instruct in Kriyāyoga, but it is for the disciple to follow his instructions whole-heartedly.

Kabīr Sat Guru ko sārā nahi, sabda na bedhā ang
Korā rahi geyā sidhrā, śādā telke sang. ***44.***

Kabīr says that the disciple who has not faithfully followed the instructions of the Master, cannot listen to the sound of

Ohmkāra, and remains where he was before initiation. He retains his own former color just as water retains its whiteness even when it is mixed with oil.

Note: The spiritual identification of the Guru and the disciple cannot be effected unless the latter practices Kriyā in complete faith and follows other instructions of the Master. It is whole-hearted surrender to Shriguru which brings ultimately man's union with the Divine.

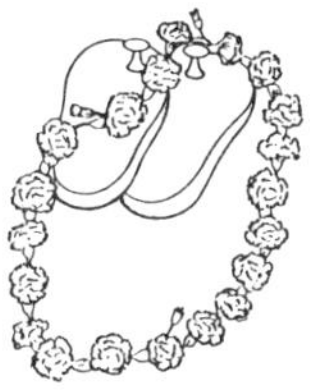

Chapter 4

Method of Worship

Kabīr danḍabat Govind Guru, avajana bando soye
Pahile bhaye parṇām tehi, nmojo āge hoye. ***1.***

Kabīr says that he used to pay obeisance to the Master who is Govinda (the Lord) Himself. Now he has no more any necessity to do it formally, for he is in a state of consciousness which keeps him constantly in an attitude of surrender.

Note: Practicing the Ohmkāra Kriyā is the spiritual method of paying obeisance to the Guru and the Paramātmā.

Kabīr jñān kathe baki baki mare, kāhe kare upādhi
Sat Guru hāmse eño kahā, sumiraṇ kara Samādhi. ***2.***

Kabīr says that people talk so much about knowledge and wisdom only in order to acquire honor and titles. But the Sadguru instructs the disciple to offer his mind to God in Samādhi.

Note: The only way to attain real knowledge and wisdom is to get absorbed in the Divine through Kriyās.

Kabīr nija sukh Rām hāy, dujā duhkha apār
Manasā vācā karmaṇā, Kabīr sumiraṇ sār. ***3.***

The proper remembrance (Sumiraṇ) of God is to live in the Divine state of consciousness. To live separated in consciousness from the Ātmā (Divine) is the cause of endless grief. To live united with Him is the proper remembrance or worship of God with mind, words and actions.

Note: To remain in the highest state of spiritual consciousness is the best service rendered to the Divine. To achieve this, a long and devoted practice of Kriyās is essential.

Bi Sumiraṇ sār hāy, āor sakal jañjal
Ādi ant sabh modhiā, dujā dekhā kāl. ***4.***

Kabīr says that it is concentration on the Divine which is all-important. Everything else is trash. The highest concentration makes one transcend past, present and future and realize Eternity Itself.

Note: "Kriyār para avasthā" is the consummation of human life devoutly to be wished. In this transcendent state of consciousness one experiences Timelessness, emancipation from the bondage of Time.

Kabīr Sumiraṇ kiyā tab janiye, tan man rahā samāy
Ādi ant madhya ek ras, bhula kabihi nā yāy. ***5.***

Practice of concentration on God with body and mind leads to an experience where everything loses its separate identity and is merged into one indescribable consciousness.

Note: Kriyās lead gradually to "Kriyār para avasthā", the Transcendent state where there is no sense of Time, no past, present or future. This state of consciousness is Joy itself.

Kabīr ādi ant madhya bhuliā pachtāoyā man māhi
Kaheñ Kabīr Hari Sumiraṇ, ohoto kiyā nāhi. ***6.***

Kabīr repents that he has not concentrated on Hari (the Divine) and therefore has not acquired the sense of Timelessness. (Kabīr here takes himself as a representative of ordinary humanity. Actually he himself is a great Saint.)

Note: The final state of spiritual consummation comes through a long practice of Kriyās.

Kabīr Sumirāṇ thoṛ hi bhālā, yau kari jāne koy
Sût na lāgi banoyāni, sahaje sabh sukh hoy. ***7.***

Kabīr says that even a little concentration is enough for a man who has known the real process of concentration. In order to weave a cloth one has to pass through difficult processes for preparing the thread. Weaving spiritual consciousness is a much more automatic and happy process.

Note: Kriyāyoga depends mainly on Prāṇāyāma or controlling the breath, and breathing is something which man is born with. Practicing Kriyā is really a much happier and easier deed than doing all sorts of worldly deeds.

Kabīr jīoban to thoṛ hi bhālā, Harikā sumiraṇ hoy
Lāk baris ki jiīunā, lekhā dhare nā koy. ***8.***

Even a small span of life with remembrance of Shri Hari (the Divine) is far better than a long life of one lakh (100,000) years spent without such remembrance.

Note: A life in which no spiritual Sādhanā is made is essentially fruitless.

Kabīr dukhme sumiraṇ sabh kare, sukhme kare nā koy
Yo sukhme sumiraṇ kare, to kāhekoñ dukh hoy. ***9.***

Kabīr says that everybody remembers the Divine while in grief, but nobody does so during happiness. If a man concentrates on the Divine during happiness, how could he ever come to grief?

Note: Generally man, engaged too much in worldly activities, neglects Kriyā, the contact with the Divine. This brings only miseries for him.

Kabīr sukhme sumiraṇ nā kiyā, dukhme kiyā yo yād
Kaheñ Kabīr tā dās ki, kñeo lāge phiriād. ***10.***

Kabīr says that one who has not remembered God in his joy, has really no claim to be heard in grief.

Note: When a man is engaged in worldly pleasures, he generally forgets the Divine. The man who performs every action with an attitude of surrender to the Divine does not become a slave to his actions. He knows that the Divine Force is the actual doer of everything and he is but an instrument. But a man steeped in worldly attachment has not cared to surrender his ego to the Divine and thus thinks himself to be the doer of his actions. Since he is the doer, who but he will suffer the fruits of his actions? He may pray to God in grief and God in His Infinite mercy will certainly grace him also, but not until he has reaped the harvest of his own deeds.

Kabīr sumiraṇ ki sudhi eoñ karo, yāyse kāmi kām
Kahe Kabīr phukāri kyāy, khusī hohiñ tab Rām. ***11.***

Kabīr says: "Remember Rāma (the Divine) with the same attachment with which a lustful person hankers after his desired object. He loudly proclaims that the Divine will be pleased at this."

Note: The word Rāma actually means One who bestows Joy. Of course the joy of union with the Divine cannot really be compared with the physical pleasure of sexual union between the lover and the beloved. Yet the union is there – between the human and the Divine consciousness. And the process through which this union is to be effected is the Kriyā. If one goes on practicing Kriyās with intense relish, he will at last reach the Transcendent state of consciousness which is Joy Absolute.

Kabīr sumiraṇ ki sudhi eoñ karo, yeño gāgari pāṇihārī.
Bole dole surtime, kahahiñ Kabīr vicāri. ***12.***

Kabīr says that when women carry pitchers full of water on their heads they move to and fro and talk among themselves. Yet, their minds are all the time fixed on the pitchers. Such is the concentration necessary for the Realization of God. Kabīr says this after a thorough consideration.

Note: The daily duties are to be done, but with our minds always concentrated on the Kûṭastha. For this a long practice of Kriyās is essential.

Kabīr sumiraṇ ki sudhi eoñ karo, yeño surabhī sut cāhi
Kahahiñ Kabīr cārācari, surabhī bācchuke pāhi. ***13.***

Kabīr says that the mother cow is grazing and eating grass in the field, and yet all the time her attention is fixed on her calf. Such is the concentration necessary for Self-Realization.

Note: We should do all our duties with our minds concentrated on the Ātmā. All work will then be transformed into worship.

Kabīr sumiraṇ ki sudhi eoñ karo, yāyse dān kāngāl
Kahahiñ Kabīr bisarai nahi, pal pal lei sabhal. ***14.***

Kabīr says that the pauper constantly hankers after gifts. In all his works he never forgets this. Such relentless hankering is what is necessary for the Realization of the Divine.

Note: The penniless pauper has to depend on the charity of others. He wants to eat good things, but cannot, because he has no money. Our concentration on God and the Guru should have the intensity of a pauper's hankering after money. But such an intensity of concentration can only be achieved through a long practice of Kriyās.

Kabīr sumiraṇ man lāgai nāhi, jagsoñ samitā yāy
Kahahiñ Kabīr suna Sādhuā, tākā kāñhā upāy. ***15.***

Kabīr says that it is very difficult to concentrate the mind which is constantly engaged in the visible world. Kabīr seems to ask a Saint: "What is the process of concentrating the mind?"

Note: Worldly attachment deviates our mind from the Ātmā. It is through the Kriyās that we have to make it steady.

Kabīr sumiraṇ señ man yab lāgai, jag soñ hoye nirāś
Kāyāko sukh choṛi key, jagsoñ hoye udās. ***16.***

Kabīr says that when actually the mind gets concentrated in the Divine, it recedes from the wordly objects, conquers the desire to have mere creature-comforts and remains above the world.

Note: When the Prāṇa-Vāyu in the "Kriyār para avasthā" settles within the head, the Sādhaka's mind drops entirely its restlessness and does not have any hankering after transitory earthly objects and mere physical happiness. With the greatest Object (viz., the Divine) in his possession he now can safely ignore the transitory earthly things.

Kabīr sumiraṇ man lāge nāhi, bikhe halāhal khāy
Kabīr hāṭ kānā rahe, kari kari thake upāy. ***17.***

Kabīr says that the mind does not like to remember God, but takes the gall of worldly enjoyments in the expectation of getting happiness. Tortured by the gall it sometimes resolves to worship God, but it neither does so nor sees any way to do it.

Note: Man, steeped in worldly attachment, sometimes takes to Kriyā, but does not generally continue it for any length of time. But apart from Kriyā, again, he cannot see any way out of his difficulties.

Kabīr sumiraṇ so man yab lāge, jñān ankuś de śis
Kaheñhi Kabīr dole nehiñ, niścay biśvās. ***18.***

Kabīr says that when actually the mind gets concentrated, it is as if the hammer of Knowledge is thrust into the head.

Note: At the "Kriyār para avasthā", Knowledge in it perfection dawns upon the devotee and the mind drops its restlessness for ever.

Kabīr sumiraṇ soñti sab bhālā, ghar ban sabhiñ ṭhāño
Kaheñ Kabīr sumiraṇ binā neha bhal ban nahiñ gāño. ***19.***

Kabīr says that for a man who concentrates on the Divine, the home and the forest are equally good places of habitation. Without remembrance of God, neither home nor forest is good.

Note: A man whose mind is concentrated in the Ātmā can adjust himself to all circumstances.

Kabīr sumiraṇ soñ siddhi hot hāy, sumirañ soñ riddhi hoy
Sumiraṇ sāñi mile, kari dekha sabh koy. ***20.***

Kabīr says that concentration on the Divine gives one 'Rddhi' as well as 'Siddhi' (success). Rddhi refers to the 8 yogic powers (aṣṭasiddhi): 'Animā' (the power of making oneself as small as an atom), 'Laghimā' (the power of becoming lighter than air), 'Byāpti' (the power of spreading oneself over the entire Universe). 'Prākāmaya' (the power to acquire anything at the mere wish). 'Mahimā' (the power to assume any shape), 'Iśitva' (the control over all beings of the Universe), 'Baśitva' (the power to move anywhere), and 'Kāmāvasāyitā' (the power to stay at any place). 'Siddhi' here means Realization of God. Kabīr asks everybody to experience it and see for himself.

Note: Kriyā leads to the Transcendent state, where, due to complete unification with the Paramātmā, the Sādhaka becomes the

Lord of the entire Universe and can have anything at the mere wish. Of course, at this stage there can be no separate wish of the devotee. His will now becomes one with the Divine will.

Kabīr sumiraṇ soñ sukh hot hāy, sumiraṇ soñ dukh yāy
Kahe Kabīr sumiraṇ kiye, sāñi māba samāy. ***21.***

Kabīr says that concentration on the Divine brings happiness and eliminates sorrow. Kabīr further says that concentration makes us merge our identity with the Lord Himself.

Note: Prolonged practice of Kriyās leads us to an exalted state of consciousness called "Kriyā para avasthā" which is full of Divine Bliss.

Kabīr sumiraṇ soñ samśay meṭe, sumiraṇ soñ meṭe śog
Kahe Kabīr sumiraṇ kiye rahe nā eko rog. ***22.***

Kabīr says that concentration on the Divine dispels doubts, disease and grief.

Note: The "Kriyār para avashtā" is a blissful state of consciousness free from doubts and disbelief, sorrow and ailments.

Kabīr sumiraṇ māhi Rāmke, ḍhil nā kijiye man
Kahe Kabīr chan ek mo, binaśī yāyegā tan. ***23.***

Kabīr says that we should not forget to concentrate on Rāma (the Lord) due to idleness, for this body may be destroyed within a moment.

Note: We should not at all drop the practice of Kriyās, for who knows when we shall have to die?

Kabīr sumiraṇ kare so śānta jan, aharniśi apne jāgi
Kahe Kabīr sumiraṇ tyaje, tāko baṛa abhāgi. ***24.***

Kabīr says that wise persons go on remembering the Divine day and night. He who does not think of God is a hapless person.

Note: Constant practice of Kriyās is the way to wisdom. A person lacking in such practice is unfortunate.

Kabīr sumiraṇ sama kuch hāy nehi, Yog yagña brat dān
Sumiraṇ sam tīrath nehi, sumiraṇ sama nāhi jñān. ***25.***

Kabīr says that nothing can be compared to concentration of the Divine – neither mere physical practice of the yogic exercises (Hathayoga, not Rājayoga which is Kriyāyoga), nor offerings in the sacred fire, nor ceremonial observance of fasting and such other religious rites, nor making gifts to others. Even a pilgrimage to a sacred place or depth of knowledge cannot be compared to the concentration in the Divine in its immediate effect of giving us liberation.

Note: The practice of Kriyās received from a Sadguru far surpasses all other religious acts in its immediacy of granting us perfect Bliss.

Kabīr jap tap sañjam Sādhan, sab sumiraṇ ko māhi
Kahe Kabīr vicāri kai sumiraṇ sam kuch nāhi. ***26.***

Kabīr says that concentration includes within itself repeating the holy names, religious practices and Self-control. Nothing, therefore, can be compared to concentration on the Divine.

Note: Kriyā includes all other practices leading to the Divine.

Kabīr sahakāmī sumiraṇ kā karei, pāoye ūcā dhām
Niha kāmī sumiraṇ kare, pāoye abical Rām. ***27.***

Kabīr says that one who remembers God with desires, reaches heaven; but one who remembers the Divine without any desire, reaches God.

Note: Kriyā is the way of concentrating on the Divine without any earthly desires. It is Kriyā which leads us to "Kriyār para avasthā", a state of complete tranquillity which is another name for Paramātmā.

Kabīr sahakāmī sumiraṇ kare, phiri āoye phiri yāy
Niha kāmī sumiraṇ kare āoyā gaman naśāy. ***28.***

Kabīr says that one who remembers God for fulfilling earthly desires has to born again and again on this earth; but one who concentrates on God without any extraneous desires, attains liberation.

Note: Kriyā practiced without desires leads to Mokṣa or liberation from the tie of Karma (Work).

Kabīr Rājā Rāṇā na baṛā, barā ye sumire Rām
Tāhi mo so jan baṛā, yo sumire nihakām. ***29.***

Kabīr says that neither the king nor the landlord is great. The great man is he who concentrates on Rāma (the Lord). But the greatest is one who constantly remembers Rāma without any earthly desires to fulfill.

Note: One who practices Kriyā only for the sake of union with the Divine is really great among men.

Kabīr sāheb kā sumiraṇ karei, tāko bando deo
Pahile āye ḍigābai, pāche lāge seo. ***30.***

Kabīr says that even gods worship the man who concentrates on the Ātmā (the Lord). The gods at first try to dissuade him, but they end by rendering him service.

Note: The sincere devotee is at first faced with many temptations to shake off his practice of Kriyā, but when he still pursues Kriyāyoga with determination, the opposition gradually gives in before his devotion.

Kabīr sumiraṇ surti lāgāike, mukh so kachuo na bol
Bāher ke paṭ dei kei, andar ko paṭ khol. ***31.***

Kabīr says that when actually the mind is concentrated in the Divine, it has no more the desire to talk. Kabīr asks to drop the screen on the outward objects, and open the screen of the inward eye.

Note: Kriyā gradually opens the inward eye till at last the devotee reaches the "Kriyār para avasthā" in which the inward and the outward become all one.

Kabīr yo bole to Ram kahi, āorehi Rām kāhāoye
Yā mukh Rām nā niklei, tā mukh pheri kāhāye. ***32.***

Kabīr says that whatever we say is the saying of Rāma (the Lord) and it is He who makes us say that. And the mouth that does not utter the name of Rāma cannot be called a mouth at all.

Note: Nothing can be said or done without the strength and consciousness granted by the Divine. Every human effort, therefore, should be conducted in an attitude of surrender to the Divine.

Kabīr mukh to soi bhalā, yā mukh niklei Rām
Yā mukh Rām nā niklei, so mukh kone kām. **33.**

Kabīr says that the mouth from which the name of Rāma comes out is good. What is the use of a mouth which does not utter 'Rāma'?

Note: Through the practice of Kriyāyoga one should be charged with the Holy Name and spirit of the Lord. Without divine consciousness human life can never reach its fruition.

Kabīr Hari kā nām me, surti rahe ek tār
Tā mukhte moti jhare, hīrā ananta apār. **34.**

Kabīr says that pearls and innumerable other jewels come out of the mouth of one who is always absorbed in the Name of Rāma.

Note: 'Kriyār para avasthā' is a state of consciousness when man becomes so identified with the Divine that every word he utters is invaluable and gives us a sense of the Illimitable.

Kabīr Hari ka nām me, bāt cālāoye āor
Tis aparādhī jīuko, tini lok nehi ṭhāor. **35.**

Kabīr says that the man who misuses the Holy Name of God, i.e., does wrong things in the Name of God, has no place in Heaven and earth, not even in the nether regions.

Note: 'Taking the Name of God' has the inner sense of 'practicing Kriyās'. One who does not practice Kriyā himself and asks others not to do it, can never be established as a Yogī. He can never attain communion with the Divine. The three worlds refer here to 'Swarga' (Heaven), 'Martya' (Earth) and 'Pātāla' (the Nether

Regions). From the Kriyā point of view 'Swarga' refers to the head (the Sahasrāra and the Ājñā Cakra), 'Martya' refers to the breast (the Anāhata Cakra) and 'Pātāla' refers to the Mūlādhāra Cakra. These three places in the body are particularly important for the Yogī in his progress towards Self-Realization.

Kabīr ratan sumiraṇī Rām ki, poe man mastul
Chabi lāgi nirakhat rahe, mit geyā Samśay śul. ***36.***

Kabīr says that the mind, while making a garland of jewels for Rāmacandra (the Lord), is blessed with a vision in which it gradually gets concentrated. All doubts are dissolved in this state of absorption.

Note: Concentration of mind in the Ājñā Cakra is the proper worship of the Lord. This has been likened to the weaving of the best garland for the Divine. Such concentration leads to innumerable visions and spiritual experiences in the Kûṭastha and leads gradually to the supreme state of consciousness where doubts torment the Sādhaka never again. The torment suffered from doubts and disbelief have been compared to the disease named Śūla, an excruciating pain in the stomach which, when it increases, reaches the heart and brings about the death of the patient.

Kabīr meri sumiraṇi Rāmki, rasanā upar Rām
Ādi yugādhi bhakti je, sabko nij biśrām. ***37.***

Kabīr says that due to constant remembrance of Rāma the Lord stays above his tongue (in the Ājñā Cakra). It is Rāma who is the origin of everything and the Master of Īṛā and Pingalā (the gangliated cords of sympathetic nerves). Absorption in him generates devotion and gradually the mind takes rest in it proper place in the Ājñā Cakra.

Note: The place of the Ājñā Cakra is above the tongue, and the 'Khecarī Mudrā' (lifting the tongue through an upward hole) practiced in Kriyāyoga makes the mind concentrated in the Ājñā Cakra. Once the mind is set at rest, the devotee experiences utter tranquillity which is Brahman Itself.

Kabīr Rām nām sumiraṇ kare, Brahmā Biṣu Maheś
Kahehiñ Kabīr sumiraṇ kare, Nārad Śukdev Śeṣ. ***38.***

Kabīr says that Brahmā, Viṣṇu and Maheśwar (the Holy Trinity symbolizing powers of Creation, Preservation and Destruction) themselves utter the Name of Rāma. Nārada (the divine sage), Śukadeva (the great sage son of Vyāsa, writer of the Mahābhārata), Śeṣa (Ananta, and indivisible part of the Lord Himself), and Kabīr himself always remain immersed in the Name of Rāma.

Note: Kriyā leads to 'Kriyār para avasthā' when the devotee with Self-Realization becomes the Self or Ātmā Itself.

Kabīr Sanakādi sumiraṇ kare. Nām Dhruba Prahlād
Jan Kabīr sumiraṇ kare, chori sakal bakbayāt. ***39.***

Kabīr says that sages like Sanaka, devotees like Dhruba and Prahlād remember Rāma (the Lord) all the time. Lovers of God do it everywhere, without wasting time in idle talks.

Note: Kriyā leads to the Transcendent stage when we remain absorbed in the experience of the Divine.

Kabīr Rām nāmke sumirte, jware patik anek
Kahe Kabīr nehi choṛiye, Rām nāmki tek. ***40.***

Kabīr says, "If you take the Name of Rāma, vile people will criticize you. But never forsake the Holy Name due to their criticism."

Note: People whose minds roam about only between the Mūlādhāra and Swādhisṭhāna, are anti-divine. Through practice of the Kriyās we must raise our minds upwards till we reach the Ājñā Cakra and then get identified with the Divine in the Sahasrāra.

Kabīr Rām nāmke sumirte, adham tare samsār
Ajāmil gaṇika Supac, seori sadan canḍār. ***41.***

Kabīr says that by taking the Name of Rāma even bad people are saved. People like Ajāmil and others turned to be great devotees by taking the Holy Name.

Note: All of us may get relieved of our sins by a devoted practice of Kriyās.

Kabīr Rām nām man lāile, yāyese pāṇi mīn
Prāṇ tyaje pal bichure, dās Kabīr kahi dīn. ***42.***

Kabīr modestly says that the devotee should concentrate his mind in the Name of Rāma, just like a fish in water.

Note: The fish cannot live except in water. So also, a human being, in order to live the proper kind of life, must always remain in Divine consciousness. This however, can only be had in "Kriyār para avasthā" for attaining which a long and devoted practice of Kriyās is essential.

Kabīr Rām nām, man lāile, yāyse nād kurang
Kahe Kabīr ṭare nehi, prān tyaje tehi sang. ***43.***

Kabīr asks the devotee to fix his mind deeply on God just as a deer fixes its mind on the sound of the flute of a hunter. The deer remains so absorbed in the sound that it does not budge an inch even when it dies.

Note: The devotee's attachment to the Divine through the Kriyās should be so deep that he will be ready to sacrifice his very life for His sake.

Kabīr Rām nām man lāile, yāyse kīṭ bhrng
Kabīr bisrāoye ābko, hoye yāy tehi rang. ***44.***

Kabīr says that as the cockroach, fascinated by the black bee, takes the color of the former, so also the devotee, absorbed in the name of Rāma, forgets himself and gets identified with him.

Note: The tradition goes that the cockroach, pursued by the black bee, is transformed into the former. So also, the devotee, by constant absorption in the Divine in the 'Kriyār para avasthā', forgets his limited bodily self, and assumes the nature of his Maker.

Kabīr Rām nām man lāile, yāyse dīp patang
Prāṇa tyaje chan ek mo, jwarata nā moṛe ang. ***45.***

Kabīr asks the devotee to concentrate his mind in the Name of Rāma just as an insect does in the burning lamp. The insect dies within a moment and yet shows no sign of pain.

Note: When the devotee enters the Divine Consciousness in the 'Kriyār para avasthā', he thinks no more of his limited self.

Kabīr Rām kahe sabh rahit hāy, tan man dhan samsār
Rām kahe bin yāt hay lāk caurāśī dhār. ***46.***

Kabīr says that by taking the Name of Rāma the devotee loses his attachment to body, mind, riches and the material world. But one who does not take the Name of Rāma has to wander through 84 *lakhs of births.

Note: Before becoming a man every being has to pass through innumerable births and deaths as lower kinds of beings. After having the human birth a man must concentrate his mind on the Divine in order to have liberation. The human being is the best of animals only because he alone has some freedom of using his own discretion. The lower animals are guided only or mainly by instincts. It is man who can turn his mind to his Maker and attain liberation or he can be anti-divine and get involved in the bondage of 'Karma' (work). Having the human birth, therefore, one should never neglect the Kriyā. It is in the Transcendent stage which can be reached only through a long practice of Kriyās that man can attain perfect tranquillity and Bliss by losing all earthly attachment.

Kabīr Rām nām ruci upje, jīu ke jwalani bujhāye
Kuhe Kabīr ek Rām nām binu, jīuke dāha nā yāye. ***47.***

Kabīr says that by developing a taste for the Name of Rāma man has all his sufferings alleviated. Without the Name of Rāma there can be no mitigation of sorrow.

Note: Concentration in the Divine through Kriyā (spiritual practices) is the only method of overcoming the seemingly endless sorrows and difficulties in human life on earth.

*** 1 lakh = a hundred thousand (1000 x 100)**

Kabīr Rām rijhāñile, jihwāso karu mat
Hari sāgar nahi bisarei, nar dekhi anant. ***48.***

Kabīr says, "Do not try to satisfy Rāma by merely uttering His Name with your tongue. Remember all the time Hari (Rāma or the Divine) who is like an endless Ocean (of Existence, consciousness and Bliss). In such a state of consciousness man knows the Infinite".

Note: We should try to achieve our union with the Divine by Sādhanā (Kriyā). By repeated practice we reach the 'Kriyār para avasthā" when we see everything as Brahman or Paramātmā.

Kabīr Rām rijhāṇile, bikh amṛt bil gāy
Phuṭā nag yo joṛiye, sayihi sandha milāy. ***49.***

When something is broken into two pieces, they can again be one if the joints of both pieces are set together. So also when Rāma is satisfied, the devotee takes everything as His manifestation, and therefore even poison is transformed into nectar for him.

Note: When the restless mind reaches the 'Kriyā para avasthā' through a long practice of Kriyās, it becomes perfectly tranquil by getting identified with the Paramātmā. In such a state of consciousness the devotee can live and move freely even in this practical world which is full of poison. Since everything has come to be Brahman for him, the bane of earthly life can no more affect him in the least.

Kabīr Rām japat kuṣṭi bhālā, cuñi cuñi paṛā cām
Kāncan deha kehi kām ki, yā mukh nāhi Rām. ***50.***

Kabīr says that even a leper with the Name of Rāma on his lips is better than a handsome person who does not utter the Holy Name.

Note: Even a diseased man who has started practicing the Kriyās is better than a healthy person without Kriyā.

Kabīr Rām japat dālidri bhālā, ṭuṭi ghar ki chān
Kāncan mandil yān de, yāñhā bhakti nahi jñān. ***51.***

Kabīr says that a poor man living in a broken hut is better if he takes the Name of Rāma than one without a devotion and wisdom living in a temple of gold.

Note: The man who has reached 'Kriyār para avasthā' has snapped his attachment to the world. Such a man is infinitely better than one who is steeped in worldly riches, without concentrating his gaze in the Kûṭastha.

Kabīr ṭāṭ oṛike Hari bhaje, tākā nām saput
Māyā eyāri makhārā, kere geye kaput. **52.**

Kabīr says that a poor man in tatters who worships Hari (Rāma, the Lord) is definitely a good son of God. On the other hand, many bad people, steeped in worldly attachment, have idly wasted their time in vulgar talks.

Kabīr sab jag nirdhanā, dhanavant nehi koye
Dhanavantā soi jāniā, yāke Rām nām dhan hoye. **53.**

Kabīr says that the entire world is poor. Nobody is rich excepting the man who has the possession of the Name of Rāma.

Note: All earthly possessions are transitory. It is only the Divine who is Eternal. The man who has reached the Divine through Kriyāyoga is therefore the only rich man, for he has attained the greatest wealth.

Kabīr Yāki gāñṭhi Rām hāy, tāko hāy sabsiddh
Karyoṛe ṭhāṛi parei āṭ siddh nao nidh. **54.**

Kabīr says that one who is in possession of the Name of Rāma has attained all siddhis (powers). The eight kinds of siddhis and nine kinds of jewels wait on him as it were with folded palms.

Note: One who has attained the 'Kriyār para avasthā' has attained all the 8 kinds of power. (See p. 41, Note on Verse 20, Chapter 4. the 8 kinds of 'siddhi' that have been described as 'Rddhi'). The 9 kinds of jewels are – gold, silver, diamond, pearl, emerald, coral, ruby, sapphire and the philosopher's stone. The Yogī can have all of them at his mere wish, although he has no desire for them.

Kabīr pargat Rām kahu, chāne Rām na gāye
Phuske ḍorā dūri karu, yo bahuri na lāgāye gāye. **55.**

Kabīr says: "Utter the Name of Rāma on your lips, if you like. But be careful that it does not disturb the Name of Rāma within. Remove the cord of whispers, for, once broken, it cannot be set right again".

Note: It is the "Anāhata Nāda" or the sound of Ohmkāra within (See p. 19) which is the real Name of Rāma or the Divine. But it is only through the practices of Kriyā that this sound can be heard continuously. If we go on whispering or chanting the Name of Rāma, the continuity of our taking the Name will be broken whenever we shall talk to others or engage our minds in some other work. It is therefore the Name within after which we should aspire.

Kabīr bāhār kāñhā dekhlāiye, antar kahiye Rām
Kaho mahaulā khalak so, parā dhanīse kām. **56.**

Kabīr says: "Let the Name of Rāma be in your mind. Why utter the same merely by mouth? What is the necessity of earning a good name in the world (by showing yourself as a virtuous man)? Your aspiration should be after the greatest, viz., God."

Note: Mere worldly recognition may bring us money. But in order to be really wealthy we have to attain the 'Kriyār para avasthā' where we reach the source of all wealth.

Kabīr nām bisāro dehako, jīyo daśā sab yāe
Yab hiñ choṛe nām ko, tab hi lāge dhāye. **57.**

Kabīr says that when a man forgets his physical self, all sorts of difficulties leave him untouched. But when he forgets the Name of Rāma, the obstacles come again.

Note: It is in the "Kriyār para avasthā" that the devotee transcends his limited self and can remain unaffected by the ups and downs of the work-a-day world. But if he leaves off practicing Kriyā, he cannot hope to attain the highest state of consciousness and so he will be liable to be upset by every danger and difficulty.

Kabīr Rām nām nahi choṛiye eha paratīta diṛ bāñdhi
Kāl kalpa byāpe nahi, ḍori nām ki sādhi. ***58.***

Kabīr says: "Never leave off the Name of Rāma. Tie yourself fast to that Name; for it is only with the cord of Name that you can expect to withstand the ravages of time".

Note: Time is a symbol of change and restlessness. Eternity transcends Time because it is changeless. Now although the human body is perishable, the human consciousness can attain the everlasting state by being one with the Divine in the "Kriyār para avasthā". But it is only by practicing Kriyā that one can reach this stage. The latent Divine Energy in the Mūlādhāra is awakened by Kriyā and is raised through the different plexuses to the Sahasrāra within the head. This linking up of the lowest with the highest cakra has been described as the Holy Chord.

Kabīr Rām hamāre māt hāy, Rām hamāre tāt
Rām hamāre mitra hāy, Rām hamāre bhrāt. ***59.***

Kabīr says that it is Rāma alone who is his mother, father, friend and brother.

Note: Since the lover of God depends on God and God alone, it is God who happens to be his mother, father, etc. Besides, in the "Kriyār para avasthā" the devotee knows that everything and everybody in this Universe is a manifestation of the Divine. Everything and everybody is God and nothing but He. (**सर्वं खल्विदं ब्रह्म**).

Kabīr Rām hamāre Āśram, Rām hamāre baraṇ
Rām hamāre jāti hāy, rahihi Rāmke śaraṇ. ***60.***

Kabīr says that Rāma is his Āśrama, Rāma is his Varṇa, Rāma is his caste. Therefore all the time he seeks the shelter of Rāma.

Note: Varṇa refers to the four great classifications of men in ancient Indian society: Brāhmaṇa, (men of Self-Realization), Kṣatriya (fighters), Vaiśya (businessmen) and Śūdra (agriculturists and service-holders). Āśrama refers to the four stages in human life in ancient India: Brahmacarya (the period of education, training and spiritual discipline), Gārhasthya (the period of life as a householder), Bānaprastha (the period of meditation in a forest or a secluded place) the Sannyāsa (the period of complete surrender to and absorption in the Divine). Caste refers to the various sub-divisions in the four Varṇas. Each of these castes, Varṇas and Āśramas had specific duties and obligations to the society. But one who is devoted to Rāma, i.e., one who practices Kriyā, transcends the limits of his own particular caste and creed, and attains complete identification with God in the "Kriyā para avasthā".

Kabīr Rām hamāre mohanī, Rām hamāre śikh
Rām hamare Iṣṭ hāy, Rām hamāre rikh. ***61.***

Kabīr says that Rāma is his enchantress, Rāma is his disciple, Rāma is his desired Deity, and Rāma is the sage for him.

Note: As one proceeds higher and higher in the path of Kriyā, one is gradually enamoured of the Divine consciousness. When at last the devotee reaches the "Kriyār para avasthā", he feels that everything is Brahman.

Kabīr Rām hamāre mantr hāy, Rām hamāre tantr
Rām hamāre auṣadhi, Rām hamāre yantr. ***62.***

Kabīr says that Rāma is his Mantra (sacred words to be repeated and meditated upon), Rāma is his Tantra (sacred Scriptures), Rāma is his medicine and Rāma is his instrument.

Note Kriyā generates complete dependence on God in all matters.

Kabīr Rām hamāre bhūmiyāñ, Rām hamāre deo
Rām hamāre sādh hāy, karhi tinhi ki seo. ***63.***

Kabīr says that Rāma is the basis of his life, Rāma is his God, and Rāma is his sādhanā. It is to Rāma that his services are offered.

Note: In the "Kriyār para avasthā" the devotee realizes that it is Divine Energy which lies latent in the Mūlādhāra, to be awakened by contact with a Sadguru. He realizes the same Paramātmā in the Sahasrāra with his practices in Kriyāyoga. The real service to the Paramātmā, therefore, is to go on practicing Kriyā, till at last we reach the "Kriyār para avasthā".

Kabīr tīrath hamāre Rām hāy, barat hamāre Rām
Dān hamāre Rām hāy, nehi āor so kām. ***64.***

Kabīr says that Rāma is his place for pilgrimage, Rāma is his sacred ceremony, Rāma is his charity. He does nothing without Rāma.

Note: Kriyā gives us the result of all sorts of good and benevolent activities. The chief aim of all such activities is to reach the Divine consciousness. Since Kriyā leads to "Kriyār para avasthā", Kriyā is the best of activities. And it is only the man who has reached the Transcendent state of consciousness ("Kriyār para avasthā") who can be a real source of well-being to man.

Kabīr monti cuni Rām hāy, Hari Hīrā O lāl
Rūpā Soṇā Rām hāy, bhojan sājan māl. ***65.***

Kabīr says that Rāma is his ruby and pearl, Rāma is his diamond and precious red stone, Rāma is his gold and silver, Rāma is his nourishment, decoration, and joy.

Note: It is in the "Kriyār para avasthā" that we reach the Paramātmā, and it is He who is our greatest treasure in life.

Kabīr soṇā rūpā kāl hāy, kankar pāthar hīr
Ek nām muktā maṇi, tāko japahi Kabīr. ***66.***

Kabīr says that gold and silver lead only to death. Diamond is nothing better than a stone-chip. The only pearl or jewel for Kabīr is the Name of God which is chanted by him.

Note: The greatest possession in life is the Lord with whom we are united in the "Kriyār para avasthā". For constantly remaining in the highest state of consciousness in the "Kriyār para avasthā", practice of Kriyās is essential.

Kabīr yab hi Ram hrday āndhāru, bhaye pāp ko nāś.
Mānukh cinigi āgko, paṛi purāṇe ghās. ***67.***

Kabīr says when Rāma rises in the heart, fear and sin are totally eliminated; just as when fire touches dry grass, the latter is completely burnt.

Note: When the Light Divine illumines our consciousness, passions fail to trouble us any longer.

Kabīr Rām yo rati ek hāy, pāp yo rati hājār
Araj rāi ghaṭ sañcare, jwāri kare sab chār. ***68.***

Kabīr says that the will of Rāma is one whereas the desires of sin are a thousand. When Rāma illumines the consciousness, all desires are burnt and driven away.

Note: In the "Kriyār para avasthā" everything is felt to be Brahman and therefore there is a feeling of oneness prevailing in the consciousness of the devotee. In such a state the innumerable diversions of the mind are completely eliminated.

Kabīr pahile burā kamāike, bāndhe biksi paṭ
Koṭi karam kāṭe palak me, yab āoye Hari oṭ. ***69.***

Kabīr says that we have made a packet of poison with so many sins formerly committed by ourselves. But when Hari (the Lord) will take us in His shelter, crores of sins will be destroyed in a moment.

Note: Long practice of Kriyās leads us to the Transcendent state of consciousness, when, due to contact with the Divine, we become absolutely good and pure.

Kabīr koṭi karma kāṭe palak me, yaño rañcak āoye nām
Anek janma yao puṇi kare, nehi nām bin thāño. ***70.***

Kabīr says: "When the Name of Rāma will be steady within yourself, the tie of even a crore of Karmas will be eliminated at once. Even your good work for many births can be of no avail. Excepting the Name (of God) there is no other way (for salvation)."

Note: The restlessness of many births can be eliminated at once as soon as we reach the "Kriyār para avasthā". It is at this stage that the Name of God settles within us forever.

Kabīr yin yin yyāysā Hari jānia, tinko tyāysā lābh
Yose bāsan bhājai, yao lāgi dhase na yāo. ***71.***

Kabīr says that every man who worships the Lord achieves realization in his own way. If you strike utensils with force, the utensils will be broken. So also if we worship Hari (the Lord) with staunch devotion, Hari destroys our body (the bodily attachment) and grants us salvation.

Note: As we go on practicing Kriyā, our contact with the Divine is intensified, till we become one with Him in the "Kriyār para avasthā". At this stage of consciousness, all bodily attachment wears off and the devotee becomes free from all bondage of desires.

Kabīr Hariko sumiri le, prāṇ yāye gā chuṭi
Gharke pacāre ādmī, calet lehi ge luṭi. ***72.***

Kabīr says: "Always remember Hari, else thy life will be lost. The thief is in thy neighborhood, ready to steal all thou hast."

Note: To remember God all the time is to stay always in the "Kriyār para avasthā". Unless one stays in this plane of consciousness the Prāṇa-Vāyu or breath cannot avoid wastage. The evils can always rob us of our rest and peace unless we remain in the Transcendent stage.

Kabīr luṭ śake to luṭ le, Rām nām hāy luṭi
Pheri pāche pachtāoge, prāṇ yāhige chuṭi. ***73.***

Kabīr says that there is an inexhaustible fund of the Name of Rāma and we may take in as much of it as we can. For once the vital breath is out, we may have to repent.

Note: While we live, we should practice as much Kriyā as possible. For unless we practice Kriyās, we cannot reach "Kriyār para avasthā"; and unless we attain "Kriyār para avasthā" before the end of this life, we shall have to be born again as a slave to attachment.

Kabīr luṭi śake to lut le, Rām nām hāy luṭi
Nām nag nike gaho nāto yāyega chuṭi. ***74.***

Kabīr says: "Take as much from the fund of Rāmanāma (the Name of Rāma) as you can. Cherish this treasure with care lest you lose it (through your fault)".

Note: We should always try to remain in the "Kriyār para avasthā."

Kabīr luṭi śake to luṭi le, Rām nām bhaṇḍār
Kāl kaṇṭh tab ghahige, rokeñ daśo duār. ***75.***

Kabīr says: "Take as much from the treasure house of Rāmanāma as you can. Shut all the ten gates of the body and hold Time steadily within your throat."

Note: There are nine gateways of our physical body through which we establish contact with the outside world – two eyes, two ears, two nostrils, the mouth, the penis and the anus. The tenth is "Brahmarandhra", a very subtle passage within the crest of the head which is opened up only after a long and devoted practice of Kriyās. For the beginner in spiritual practices all the nine doors are shut for the time being when he practices the "Yonimudrā" (to be learned from the Sadguru), the Kriyā in which the Sādhaka is required to withdraw his attention from the outside world and fix his gaze in the Kûṭastha by concentrating on the middle point in between the eyebrows. But for the Yogī who has attained "Kriyār para avasthā" and has also the tenth gate open, it is not necessary that he should shut any of the gates by closing his eyes and other related practices. Even when they remain open, the devotee at this stage is absorbed in the Divine (the Rāmanāma referred to by Shri Shri Kabīr). His Prāṇa-Vāyu is always within the Suṣumnā and therefore the restlessness of Time is no more felt by him. By being one with the Divine, his consciousness, too, becomes Timeless, Eternal.

Kabīr Rām nām japi lijlye, choṛi jīu ki vāṇī
Pariśme biti gei, soi, āpu par jāni. ***76.***

Kabīr says: "Go on taking the Name of Rāma, without paying any heed to what people say (against it). While Time is being wasted in vain, we are still making differences between ourselves and others."

Note: We should go on practicing Kriyā till we reach "Kriyār para avasthā" when we realize the essential oneness of all beings. Only then can we "do to others" as we "would be done by".

Kabīr Rām nām nidhi lijiye, tyaji māyā bikh boj
Bār bār nehi pāiye, mānukh janam ki moj. ***77.***

Kabīr says: "Shake off the poisonous burden of Māyā (worldly attachment) and take up the jewel of the Name of Rāma; for you may not have the chance of having the human birth again and again."

Note: Since the human body is best suited for Sādhanā, it is the primary duty of every human being to go on practicing Kriyā till he reaches the "Kriyār para avasthā."

Kabīr Rām nām japi lijiye, yab lagi diyā bāti
Tel ghāṭe bāti bujhei, tab śogrā din rāti. ***78.***

Kabīr says: "Go on taking the Name of Rāma, for the wick of the lamp (of life) is being dried up. As soon as the oil (the breath) is exhausted, the light will be extinguished. At that time your days will be as dark as night."

Note: We should go on practicing Kriyā so long as we have breath.

Kabīr śutā keyā kare, jāgi nā japei Murāri
Ek dinbhi choṛ nā, lambe pāo pasāri. ***79.***

Kabīr says: "What use lying down (in idleness) now? The day will come when you will have to lie down stretching your legs (i.e., when you will die). Keep yourself awake at present and go on taking the Name of Murāri (the Lord)."

Note: We should practice Kriyā in order to awake in Divine Consciousness.

Kabīr śutā keyā kare, uṭhi keño nā roe dukh
Yākā bāsā gor me, so keño śoe sukh. ***80.***

Kabīr says: "Why are you lying down? What happiness can there be for a man whose habitation is actually within the grave? Why does he not arise and weep?"

Note: Since death is ready to snatch us away from life any moment, we should try to reach the deathless eternal consciousness by constantly practicing Kriyās.

Kabīr śutā keñā kare, guṇ Govindkā gāo
Tere śir par Yam khāṛā, kharac dei keyā khāo. ***81.***

Kabīr says: "How could anybody lie down without any anxiety when Yama (the god of death) is just on his head? Let him sing the glory of Govinda (the Lord). How did you eat (use) the provision (granted by the Lord)?"

Note: We all have received from the Divine the ability to practice Kriyā (sing the glory of God), and we should make the best use of it.

Kabīr śutā keyā kare, śute hoy akāj
Brahmako āsan tigā, śoyat kāl ki lāj. ***82.***

Kabīr says: "Why lie down and sleep? If you waste your time in idleness, you will be separated from the Brahman (the Divine) within yourself and thus allow yourself to be devoured up by Time."

Note: To practice Kriyā is to achieve God-contact for ourselves. To drop the practice is to be troubled by the fear of death and all sorts of anxieties.

Kabīr śutā keyā kare, kāhe na dekhai jāgi
Yāke sang so bichurā, tāhike sang lāgi. ***83.***

Kabīr says: "No purpose can be served by resting in idleness. Awake and see that you so long lost your contact with the Divine. Try to regain the same."

Note Kriyā is the way to have contact with the Divine within ourselves. We should therefore shake off our idleness in practicing the Kriyā received from the Sadguru.

Kabīr nid niśāni nic ki, uṭha Kabīrā jāgi
Āor rasāyan choṛke, tom Rām rasāyan lāgi. ***84.***

Kabīr says that (excessive) sleep is the sign of a lower stratum of consciousness. He asks himself to rise up and take the best medicine, viz., Rāma, leaving all other medicines.

Note: Lack of practice in Kriyās keeps our mind at the lower centres of our body. If our mind is lost (thoroughly absorbed) in the Divine within the Sahasrāra in the "Kriyār para avasthā", we reach the summum bonum of life. This highest state of consciousness is the perfect cure for all kinds of earthly maladies.

Kabīr āpne pāhare jāgiye, rahiye nehi śoye
Nā jāno chin ek mo, keskā pāhārā hoye. ***85.***

Kabīr says: "Keep awake and be your own watchman. Don't sleep. Who knows who will be your watchman the very next moment?"

Note: Kriyā is the way to achieve Self-consciousness. It is in the "Kriyār para avasthā" that we are our own masters. Lack of God-contact (through Kriyā) makes us slaves to our passions.

Kabīr śoyā so niphal geyā, jāge so phal lei
Sāheb hak nā rākhei, yab mānge tab dei. ***86.***

Kabīr says that lying down in idleness is fruitless, but keeping awake brings us the desired result. The Lord never withholds from us our reasonable dues. He grants them whenever we pray for them.

Note: The greatest reward in human life is Self-Realization, which is another name for God-Realization. For achieving this reward man must be up and doing with the Kriyās received from his spiritual Master.

Kabīr keso kahi kahi kuhu kiye, śoiyenā pāo pasāri
Rāti dio saphā kuhu kanā, kabuhu ke lāge gohāri. ***87.***

Kabīr says: "Whom should I ask repeatedly, 'What have you been doing?' Do not lie down stretching you legs. Work day and night. Who knows when the call will come?"

Note: Unless we keep our consciousness awake with Kriyās, we cannot hear the call of the Divine, viz., the Anāhata Nāda or Ohmkāra.

Kabīr yāyse man māya rame, tyāse Rām ramāye
Tārā manḍal choṛike, yāñhā ke so tāñhā yāye. ***88.***

Kabīr says that if the mind is absorbed in Rāma in the same manner in which it gets absorbed in earthly attachment, it will reach the same consciousness from where it originated. Kabīr advises the devotee to leave off attachment to the cluster of stars (i.e., earthly titles and possessions).

Note: Kriyā lifts our minds gradually from attachment to earthly titles, riches and other possessions to the Divine in the "Kriyār para avasthā."

Kabīr jāgat śoyat Rām kahu, pare utāne Rām
Uṭhat baiṭhat Rām kahu, pāot añcoyat Rām. ***89.***

Kabīr says: "Take the Name of Rāma while awake or asleep, while rising or sitting, while taking meals or washing you hands after the meals."

Note: Prolonged practice of Kriyās leads us to a state of consciousness when we spontaneously remain united with the Divine. In such a state of consciousness the external organs of our body may go on doing all sorts of duties while the mind remains in God-contact. This is the state reached by Sadgurus or Saints.

Kabīr kṣudhā kāli kukurī, kare bhajan me bhanga
Oyāko ṭukurā ḍārike, sumiraṇ karo nihśanka. ***90.***

Kabīr says that Hunger is like a black bitch who disturbs Sādhanā. Give her, therefore, some food and remember God without fear.

Note: The path of Kriyā leads us gradually to non-attachment. Since it is impossible to drop all earthly desires at once, we have to satisfy them to some extent in honest ways. It is only in the "Kriyār para avasthā" that perfect non-attachment is possible.

Kabīr grhīkā ṭukrā apac hāy, tāke lambe dānt
Bhajan kare to ubare, nahi to phāṛe ānt. ***91.***

Kabīr says that the food of a householder is not digested, for he has long teeth, i.e., he earns his money generally by various misdeeds. Such a man can only be saved by worshipping God. Otherwise, his intestines are cut off (i.e., he comes only to misery).

Note: For the expiation of sins already committed for earning his livelihood, the householder should go on practicing Kriyās.

Kabīr girihī keri madhukari, khāi rahe yo soi
Kaheñ Kabīr sumiraṇ binā, ant duheli hoi. ***92.***

Kabīr says that the mendicant who collects his rice (or other foodstuffs) from the house of a family-man should always remember the Divine. Otherwise the fruits of his virtuous actions are lost.

Note: The householders do not always earn money by virtuous means. Therefore to neutralize the sins associated with the gifts from householders, the mendicant should always go on practicing Kriyas.

Kabīr Govindke guṇ gāote, kabhu nā kijiye lāj
Āb padavī āge mukti, ek pantha dui kāj. ***93.***

Kabīr says: "Never feel ashamed to praise Govinda (the Lord). This will first of all give you a good name, and later on, salvation. Thus you will catch two birds at one stroke."

Note: If the devotee goes on sincerely practicing Kriyās, he will earn a good name by being a good man, and gradually reach "Kriyār para avasthā".

Kabīr guṇ gāye guṇha kāṭe, rate Rām viyog
Ahiniśi Hari dhyāoye nahi, mile nā durlabh yog. ***94.***

Kabīr says that if the devotee sings in praise of God, all his defects are rectified. But unless he meditates upon Shri Hari (the Lord) all the time, how could there be the rare union (between the devotee and the Lord)?

Note: Kriyā gradually eliminates our dirt and dross. But the highest union with the Divine can only be achieved in the "Kriyār para avasthā".

Kabīr kaṭhinai khari, yo sumarei Harinām
Śuli upar khelnā, girei to nāhi ṭham. ***95.***

Kabīr says that it is of course difficult to go on taking the Name of Hari, for if somebody has to play (show gymnastic feats) on a śūla (a sharp rod which can pierce the whole body), he has to be very cautious; for once he falls, it is death for him.

Note: Kriyā is like playing on the spinal cord. Unless it is done with proper devotion, egoism might develop and stand in the way of the final spiritual fulfillment of the Sādhaka.

Kabīr lambā mārag duri ghar, bikaṭ pantha bahu bhār
Kahe Kabīr keño pāiye, dulabh Hari didār. ***96.***

Kabīr says that the path is long, the home is far off, the way is full of fears and the pilgrim has a heavy burden on his back. How could he achieve union with the rare Hari (the Lord) under the circumstances?

Note: There are many obstacles on the path of Kriyā. Sometimes the devotee misuses the spiritual powers that gradually come to him through the Kriyās. Sometimes he even sees hideous figures in his Kûṭastha. But if the devotee still goes on with his Sādhanā with a complete surrender to his Shriguru, the difficulties will gradually pass off and he will reach the "Kriyār para avasthā".

Kabīr Harike milanki, bāt śuni hām doye
Ki kachu Harikā Nām le, ki kara ūcā hoye. ***97.***

Kabīr says: "I have heard about two kinds of union with Shri Hari: one is by taking His Name and another by staying in the highest state of consciousness."

Note: There are two kinds of union with the Divine: One is by practicing Kriyās and the other by staying in the "Kriyār para avasthā".

Kabīr āñkhṛiāñ jhāñipaṛi, pantha nihāri
Jibṛl āñchālā paṛe, Rām pukāri pukāri. ***98.***

Kabīr says: "By constantly gazing on the path my eyes have become dimmed, and by constantly crying Rāma my tongue has been exhausted".

Note: It is very difficult to continue the practice of Kriyās in the face of many physical and mental obstacles. But constant surrender to the Sadguru leads us at last to the desired goal.

Kabīr nayanhune jhari laiyā, ramhaṭ bahe niśi yām
Papihā yeño piyā piyā kare, kabre milenge Rām. ***99.***

Kabīr says: "Just as the bird pāpihā goes on crying 'O dearest', so also should you call Rāma (the Lord) throughout the days and nights with tears in your eyes."

Note: A devoted practice of Kriyās will increase the yearning of the Sādhaka for getting united with the Divine in the "Kriyār para avashtā".

Kabīr cintā cingi uṛiā, cahudiś lāgi lāiye
Hari sumiraṇ hāthe ghaṛā, beghi lahu bujhāye. ***100.***

Kabīr says that sparks of the fire of anxiety are everywhere in the air. But the devotee has in his hand the water pitcher in the form of remembrance of Shri Hari, with the help of which he will be able to put the fire out.

Note: One is relieved of all anxieties if one practices Kriyā with devotion.

Kabīr cintā to Harinām ki, āor na citoye dās
Yo kichu cītoye Nām binu, soi kāl ki phāñs. ***101.***

Kabīr says that the only thought worthwhile is that of the Name of Hari. Other thoughts are entirely useless. Whatever we think except the Name of the Divine, will only lead us to death.

Note: To stay in the "Kriyās para avasthā" is salvation. The rest is bondage.

Kabīr swapnema barbarāike, jore kahegā Rām
Oyāke pagki paitari, mere tanko cām. ***102.***

Kabīr says that a man who cries aloud the name of Rāma even in his dreams is so great that the soles of his feet are fit to be the skin of Kabīr's body.

Note: Kabīr is so modest that he considers himself to be a servant of those who are always absorbed in the Divine, always in the "Kriyār para avasthā."

Kabīr nimikhi nimirānu kijliye, ûr antar so Rām
Kahahi Kabīrā Rām kahu, sakal sañoyāre kām. ***103.***

Kabīr says: "See Rāma within yourself and without, with winkless eyes. If you do this, all your desires will be fulfilled."

Note: It is in the highest Samādhi, in the "Kriyār para avasthā" that the mind becomes absolutely calm and the body motionless. It is this absorption in the Divine which brings consummation to the devotee.

Kabīr bhajan kareta bhaje sabhe, guṇ indri cit cor
Sar pantha candan parihari, yab caṛi bole mor. ***104.***

Kabīr says that people worship God, but their hearts are stolen by the different properties of Māyā (the three Guṇas of Sattva, Rajas and Tamas) and the sense-organs. It is for this reason that they cannot see God. Snakes find shelter in the sandalwood forest, but as soon as the peacock comes, they are at once driven out. Similarly, with the Realization of the Divine, the enemies of man's spiritual success take to their flight at once.

Note: The world of Nature is characterised by three kinds of properties which are called Guṇas. They are Sattva (propensity towards calmness and tranquillity), Rajas (propensity towards restlessness, perseverance in earthly desires and their fulfillment), Tamas (idleness, inertia). It is only in the "Kriyār para avasthā" that man transcends all these Guṇas and attachment to the body with all its organs. But once we transcend them, the Divine in all His glory will be revealed to us. The comparison with a peacock has a special point about it. The plumes of a peacock are a variegated colors. So also the vision of the Divine in the Kûṭastha (visible through "Yonimudrā" due to the grace of Shriguru) is full of varied shades of color.

Kabīr śwās suphal soi jāniye, Harikā sumiraṇ lāye
Āor śwās ehuñ gayā, kari kari bahut upaye. ***105.***

Kabīr says that only that breath is fruitful which is engaged in meditating Shri Hari. All other breaths, however engaged in various kinds of work, are useless.

Note: It is only in the "Kriyār para avasthā" that the breath is united with Brahman. We should therefore go on practicing Kriyās in order to reach that state.

Kabīr yāki puñji śwās hāy, chin āoye chin yāye
Tāko yāysā cāhiye, rahe Rām lolāye. ***106.***

Kabīr says that men have the only stock-in-trade, viz., breath. But even that is constantly restless–coming and going alternately. Hence we should always be absorbed in the Divine (for, it is only then that the breath becomes motionless and steady).

Note: It is because the Prāṇa-Vāyu (breath) is restless that our minds too are restless. Unless we can control our breath by Prāṇāyāma, our minds cannot be concentrated. Hence it is absolutely necessary that we should practice Kriyās.

Kabīr kāñhāñ bharosā dehako, binaśī yāye sin māhiñ
Śwās śwas sumiraṇ kare, āor upāy kachu nāhi. ***107.***

Kabīr says that we cannot at all depend on the body, for it may be destroyed any moment. Hence there is no other way but to think of God in every breath.

Note: Controlling the breath by Kriyā will not only increase the longevity of the body by arresting its wastage, it will also lead us to Self-Realization in the "Kriyār para avasthā".

Kabīr ajapā sumiraṇ ghaṭ bīce, dinho śiri śiri janihār
Tāhi so man lāile, kahahiñ Kabīr vicār. ***108***

Kabīr after much deliberation, says that if man constantly engages his mind in the meditation of Ohmkāra, he will experience an indefinable bliss which is Brahman.

Note: The aim of the devotee should be to attain the Transcendent state of consciousness of "Kriyār para avasthā". For this, however, a steady practice of Kriyās is essential.

Kabīr ajapā sumiraṇ hot hāy, kaho śānt kohi ṭhaur
Kar jihwā sumiraṇ kare, eha sabh manki dauṛ. ***109.***

Kabīr says that "ajapā" meditation (i.e., absolute concentration in the Divine, "Kriyār para avasthā") is the only shelter for Saints. Taking the Name of God with tongue or the beads and fingers cannot lead one very far, for it is merely a movement of the mind.

Note: It is Kriyā which gradually leads one to utter Tranquillity and Bliss.

Kabīr ajapā sumiraṇ hot hāy, śunya maṇdal asthān
Kar jihwā tāñhā nā cale, man pangul tāñhā yān. ***110.***

Kabīr says that "ajapā" meditation leads us to the "Śūnyamandal" (the seemingly empty space within the Sahasrāra), the seat of the Paramātmā within our body. Fingers or the tongue can never reach there. Even the mind has no power to reach that place.

Note: It is only in the "Kriyār para avasthā", when our breath becomes motionless that we reach God.

Kabīr mālā kaṭki, bahut jan kari pher
Mājā pher śwās ki, yāme gāñṭhi nāhi sumer. ***111.***

Kabīr says: "Do not count the wooden beads; take to the beads of breath which will offer you no knotty resistance (as in the wooden beads)".

Note: Prolonged practice of Kriyās will lead us to our consummation.

Kabīr man mālā Satguru dei, paon surtite poe
Binu hāte niśidin phire, Brahma jap tāñhā hoye. ***112.***

Kabīr says: "The Sadguru has indicated the mind as the beads. Join your mind to your breath, day and night, irrespective of counting beads with your hands. Then and then alone you will reach Brahman (The Absolute)."

Note: Kriyā is the process of uniting our mind with the Prāṇa-Vāyu and leading it gradually to the higher cakras (plexuses) till it reaches the Ājñā Cakra (within the forhead) and then gets lost in the Sahasrāra by being united with the Supreme consciousness in the "Kriyār para avasthā". The most proper "japa" (taking any of the Names of God) is therefore no outward process, but being united with the breath. This is called "ajapā".

Kabīr māiājap nā kar jap, mukhte kaha nā Rām
Man merā Sumiraṇ kare, māy pāye biśrām. ***113.***

Kabīr says: "Do not take the Name on the beads or the fingers or with the tongue. My mind is meditating, and therefore I have attained rest".

Note: Prolonged practice of Kriyās leads the mind to absorption and identification with the Divine. When there is no separate existence of the mind, there is no separate existence of the human consciousness in the devotee. This is what is described as rest by Kabīr. And this state of rest can only be attained in the "Kriyār para avasthā".

Kabīr mālā to karme phire, jihwā phire mukh māhi
Manuā to caudiś phire, iyeto sumiraṇ nāhi. ***114.***

Kabīr says that when the rosary moves along the fingers and the tongue moves within the mouth, the mind, too, roams about in all four directions. This can never be called remembrance of the Divine.

Note: Unless the mind, through Kriyās, is concentrated in the Divine, no outward action can be called real worship.

Kabīr Rām nāmkā sumiraṇ, hāñsi kare bhau khijh
Ulṭā sulṭā nipje, yāseñ kṣet kā bīj. ***115.***

Kabīr says that the man who is always absorbed in the meditation of Rāma is ridiculed by others. But such ridicule does not make any material difference for him. When the seeds are sown in a field, their mouths do not always remain upwards. But when the seeds germinate, their mouths are always upwards and the roots downwards. So also, the Saintly person, however much he might live amidst worldly men and however much they might try to upset him, has always his mind towards the Divine.

Note: People with worldly attachment are not always able to realize the greatness of a man who is absorbed in the Divine, and as such they often try to upset his tranquillity. But the man who is in the "Kriyār para avasthā" cannot really be upset.

Kabīr sumiraṇ māha lāgai de, surti āpni śoye
Kahati Kabīr sāmsār guṇ, tujhe nā byāpe keye. ***116.***

Kabīr says: "Engage your mind in the remembrance (of the Divine). In that state the mind will not go anywhere else; it will rather remain automatically concentrated, and worldly attachment will not be able to exert its influence upon you."

Note: Once the devotee attains the "Kriyār para avasthā", his mind will never stoop down to earthly attachment.

Kabīr sumiraṇ surti so, hot rahat hāy mor
Ahuṭ mukh sumiraṇ kare, ahiniśi kai karor. ***117.***

Kabīr says: "My mind is always engaged in the remembrance of God and therefore my mouth is taking the Name millions of times during a single day and night."

Note: Uttering the Name of God by mouth takes time. But when we always remain in the "Kriyār para avasthā", it is not necessary to utter the Name separately, because the mind is always engaged in it. Such constant concentration is equal to taking the Name of God innumerable times.

Kabīr rag rag bole Rāmajī, rom rom ra ramkār
Sahajei dhuni lāgi rahe, kahanhi Kabīr vicār. ***118.***

Kabīr says after much deliberation that each of his nerves is uttering "Rāma" and every pore of his skin is uttering 'Ohm'. These sounds rise automatically within his own body.

Note: A long practice of Kriyās gives rise to the 'Anāhata Nāda', the 'Ohmkāra' in its endless varieties, and keeps the Sādhaka (devotee) absorbed all the time. The sounds, however, are completely internal and continue within the body.

Kabīr sahaj hi dhuni lāgi rahe, set ehu ghaṭ māhiñ
Hirde Hari Hari hot hāy, mukhki hājati nāhi. ***119.***

Kabīr says: "Since the 'Anāhata' sound is always there within the heart, since the Name of Hari already resides there, what necessity is there to utter the same loudly?"

Note: In the "Kriyār para avasthā" the devotee remains constantly absorbed in the Divine.

Kabīr pāñc saki piu piu kare, chaṭā sumir man
Āi surti Kābīr ki, pāyā Rām Ratan. ***120.***

The five female friends (meaning the five senses) are constantly hankering after their dearest (viz., the Ātmā, the Divine) and the sixth viz., the mind, is always meditating on Him. It is under these circumstances that Kabīr has obtained the invaluable Jewel who is Rāma (the Lord).

Note: In the highest state of consciousness ("Kriyār para avasthā") all our sense-organs and the mind are always concentrated in the Divine and perform all activities from that level.

Kabīr merā man sumire Rām ko, merā man Rāmahi āhi
Āpne Rāmahi hoy, śis noyāyoñ kāhi. ***121.***

Kabīr says that by constantly meditating on Rāma, his mind itself has become Rāma. To whom, therefore, would he bow down his head?

Note: Due to complete identification with God in the "Kriyār para avasthā" the devotee has no separate consciousness on the finite human level. He becomes one with the Infinite, the Supreme Self.

Kabīr tu tu karte tu bhāyā, mujhme rahi nahu
Oyāroñ tere nām par, jit dekhti ta tuñ. ***122.***

Kabīr says: "By constantly thinking of 'You' (God), I have come to be You Yourself. O! The Glory of Your Name! To whichever direction I turn my gaze, I find You alone." (There are no more two, but One. Even there is nobody to say that there is only One).

Note: In the "Kriyār para avasthā" everything in this universe is felt to be Brahman and nothing else.

Kabīr tu tu karte tu bhayā tujhme rahe samāy
Tomhiñ māhi mil rahā, āb man anat na yāy. ***123.***

Kabīr says: "By always meditating upon You I have become You. I am in You and I have been united with You. Therefore my mind does not move elsewhere".

Note: A long practice of Kriyās makes us absolutely concentrated in the Divine in the "Kriyār para avasthā".

Kabīr sumiraṇ choṛike, pal yo bāhar yāye
Kaheñ Kabīr sumiraṇ binā kaho kāñhā ṭhaharāye. ***124.***

Kabīr says that without meditation on God the mind can never be concentrated and still even for a moment.

Note: Excepting the "Kriyār para avasthā" the mind can never completely drop its restlessness and be absolutely calm and concentrated.

Kabīr kahetā yāt hoṇ śuntā hāy sab koye
Rām kahe kal hoyegā, nehi to bhāla nā hoye. ***125.***

Kabīr says: "Everybody (Every Saint) has said and everybody has heard that all good can be acheived by taking the Name of the Lord (by meditation) and only the opposite is possible if we do not take His Name (i.e., if we do not concentrate our minds in Him)".

Note: The Sadguru tells everybody that to practice Kriyās is the source of all that is really good and beneficial, for it is by practicing Kriyās that we can attain "Kriyār para avasthā", the only state of consciousness free from all anxiety and full of Bliss.

Kabīr bhāli bheñyi Hari bichreye, śirki geyi bālāi
Hām yyāyse rahe, āb kuch kāhi nā yāye. ***126.***

Kabīr says: "It is good that I have forgotten now to take the Name of Hari. The burden on my head has now been completely off. Now I have become my real Self. It is no more possible to describe the state of consciousness I am in."

Note: When the devotee is constantly in the "Kriyār para avasthā", he has no more any necessity (excepting, of course, for the good of others) to practice Kriyās. By "taking the Name of God" we are to mean "practicing Kriyās". The aim of Kriyā is to achieve union with the Divine. If that union is achieved once and for all, the devotee becomes the Lord Himself in his consciousness. What use remains for him now of the Kriyās? The Kriyā is for the aspirant. The "Kriyā para avasthā" is the goal.

Kabīr jan Kabīr bandan kare, kis bidhi kijiye seo
Oyār pār ki gami nehi, tu man man manij deo. ***127.***

Kabīr says that devotees (his disciples) want to serve him and ask him the process of rendering service. Kabīr wants to tell them that service to the Infinite can be done only by offering your entire mind to Him (i.e., by concentrating your mind in Him and Him alone). Otherwise who will be the servant and who the Master (since everything is Brahman)?

Note: The most proper worship of the Divine is to be identified with Him in the "Kriyār para avasthā".

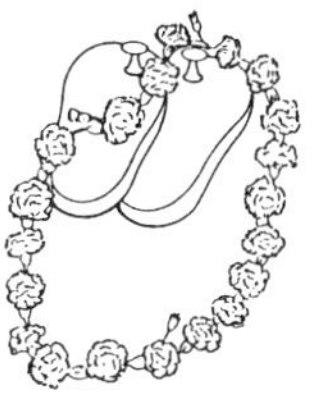

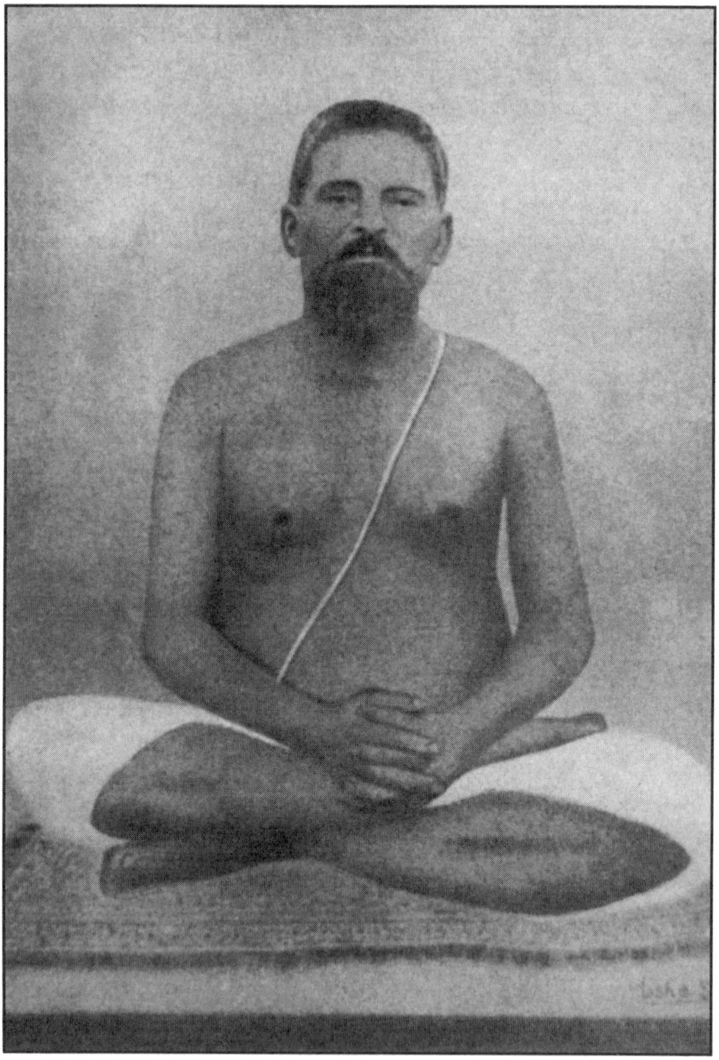

Yogacharya Shrimat Panchanan Bhattacharya

Advent: November, 1853 A.D. Mahasamadhi: August 24, 1919 A.D.

Chapter - 5

On Wisdom

Kabīr ākil araśteñ utari, bīdhinā dinho bāñṭī
Ek abhāgā rahi gayā, ekanha liyā sughāṭi. ***1.***

Kabīr says that the Lord has distributed the sense of right and wrong which has come down from Him equally amongst all. But Kabīr has remained a hapless person (really, a person who has transcended fate), for he is satisfied with one beautiful ghaṭ (bathing place in a tank or river).

Note: We have of course inherited our sense of right and wrong from the Creator, but it is only when we become identified with Him that we transcend earthly right and wrong and enter the zone of "All Right". This can only be done in the "Kriyār para avasthā". At this stage we do not do any work according to the common laws of right and wrong. Since we surrender our ego completely at the Feet of God and get merged in Divine Consciousness, we do not have to suffer the fruits of our deeds. Kabīr has attained such a state of consciousness. By a beautiful bathing 'ghaṭ' he means Divine Consciousness in which he can take his dip.

Kabīr yas panchī bankhan parā, suā ke buddhi nāhiñ
Ākil bihunā mānoyā, eo bandhā jaga māhiñ. ***2.***

Kabīr says that as a bird without wisdom is caught and put into a cage, so a man without wisdom is put within the cage of life and death.

Note: Wisdom proper can only be attained in the "Kriyār para avasthā" and it is only at this stage that one can attain complete liberation from the bondage of 'Karma', the bondage one must suffer from one's good or bad deeds. Even good deeds bring about bondage when they are done with earthly attachment and desires. Since the individual in ordinary life thinks that this or that is his own doing, the results of his deeds, good or bad, come upon him. But a man who after prolonged practice of Kriyās, has transcended his limited self and has become one with the Self Supreme, knows that he does nothing. Everything has been done by Divine Will. Hence he becomes free from the law of 'Karma', since all responsibility has now devolved on God Himself.

Kabīr binā osil cākri, binā ākil ki deñha
Binā jñān kā Yogiā, phir lāgāye kheha. ***3.***

A Yogī without realization is like employment without payment or body without intelligence. Such men have to born again and again.

Note: It is only in the "Kriyār para avasthā" that a man has liberated consciousness. Only in such a state he goes beyond the law of Karma and becomes perfectly free from the cycle of birth and death. [Of course even such a man may be born again on earth, but then, he easily becomes a Saint and saves many people from sins.]

Kabīr jal paroyāṇe machri, ghaṭ paroyāṇe buddhi
Yāko yyāysā Guru milā, tāko tyāysā śuddhi. ***4.***

Kabīr says that as fishes vary according to the varying depths of water, and as intelligence varies in different kinds of bodies, so also the purity of consciousness varies according to the capabilities of the spiritual Guide (the Guru).

Note: The purity of consciousness grows according to the intensity of practicing Kriyās. Complete purity can only be attained in the "Kriyār para avasthā", when we become indentified with Brahman. For achieving this state, however, we must receive the Grace of a Guru who has himself become identified with the Divine.

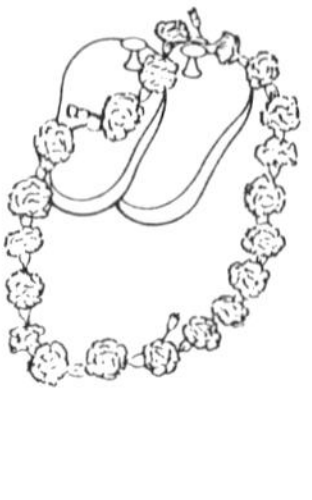

Chapter - 6

On Sadguru's Instructions

Kabīr Hariji ehi vicāriā, sākhi kañhe
Kabīr Bhao Sāgarme jīb hāy, śunī kai lāge tīr. ***1.***

Kabīr says after much deliberation that Shri Hari (the Lord) is the Eternal witness (to all our activities). That men lie immersed in the Ocean of births and deaths, is a cause of pain for the Maker, a pain like that caused by a piercing arrow.

Note: The Sadguru is the representative of God. He feels for the miserable condition of his disciples and leads them, through Kriyā, to the "Kriyār para avasthā", the Supreme state of Consciousness in which alone they can have absolute tranquillity and freedom from bondage.

Kabīr kāl kāl tatkāl hay, burā nā kahiye koye
An bowoye so dāhiṇo, bowoye so lūntā hoye. **2.**

Kabīr says that Time (Eternity) is Brahman, and nobody can blame Him. When somebody sows the seeds, he himself must reap the harvest. (He must enjoy or suffer the fruits of his own deeds.) But the man who does not sow any seeds (i.e., does not do any work with egotistic attachment), becomes free from bondage (of good and evil results).

Note: It is because man is not generally free from earthly attachment or desires, that he has to suffer the results of his deeds and has to be born again and again in order to reap the harvest of his own doings, good or evil. But attachment or desire is caused by the restlessness of mind. It is to the restless mind that Eternal Time seems to be a fractional, ever-changing flow. When, through Kriyās, a man reaches the completely tranquil state, he is said to have reached the Eternity. It is then that his mind is merged in the Divine and has no restlessness, no desires.

Since at this stage the individual loses his separate ego, his will becomes one with the Universal Will and his self is liberated from all kinds of bondage. To such a Saint remaining in the "Kriyār para avasthā", there can be no conventional distinction between good and evil, because everything for him has been submerged in the One Absolute good, viz., Brahman. It is only such a man who can be said to have an absolute surrender to the Divine, which is another name for complete identification of consciousness with Him.

Kabīr yo toko kāñṭā boye, tāko boro tuñ phul
Toko phulkā phul hāy, oyāko hāy triśul. ***3.***

Kabīr says: "Offer flowers to the man who offers you thorns. Your flowers are really flowers, but his thorns will be like a trident destroying himself".

Note: The disturbance caused by worldly people to the practice of Kriyās is like thorns. But the devotee should yet inspire them to get initiated into Kriyāyoga. Those who still refuse to practice Kriyās will come to difficulties. (The three prongs of a trident can be taken as Īṛā, Pingalā and Suṣumnā – the three main channels through which the Prāṇa-Vāyu flows inside the human body. Of course, it is the Suṣumnā – the very delicate passage within the spinal cord through which the Prāṇa-Vāyu must flow for leading us to Divine Consciousness.)

Kabīr kahete ko kahi yān de, unhaki buddh mat-i lehu
Sākaṭ āo puni śoyan ko, pheri jabāb mat-i dehu. ***4.***

Kabīr says: "Do not accept the views of those who indulge in mere useless words. Let them say whatever they like. Do not listen to them. Let them bark like dogs. Give them no reply."

Note: The devotee should stick to practicing Kriyās without paying any heed to the vain words of materialistic people.

Kabīr haśtī caṛāye jñānke, sahaj dolecā dāri
Śoyanrūp samsār hāy, bhukan de jhakmārī. ***5.***

Kabīr says: "Spread the cover of Sādhanā on the back of the elephant, and place Realization on it. People will bark like dogs without any rhyme or reason; but let them go on. They cannot do any harm to you."

Note: The devotee in the "Kriyār para avasthā" remains concentrated within the Sahasrāra which is compared to an elephant. The Prāṇa-Vāyu may be likened to the seat on the back of the elephant, because it is with the help of the Prāṇa-Vāyu that the devotee reaches his spiritual height. Once he attains his consummation, he no more cares for public applause or condemnation.

Kabīr gārite sabh upje, kāl kaṣṭa āru mic
Hāri cale so sādhu hāy, lāgi mare so nīc. ***6.***

Kabīr says that all sorts of mishaps might ensue from quarrels and abuses – bloody feuds or at least great mental pain. Sages, therefore, do not indulge in quarrels. They rather accept defeat of their own accord. It is only the lower sort who engage themselves in useless conflicts.

Note: Men who are in the "Kriyār para avasthā" have neither the time nor the inclination to pursue a quarrel.

Kabīr kahe myāy kyā kahoñ, thāke Brahmā Maheś
Rām Nām tatu sār hāy, sabh kāhu upadeś. ***7.***

Kabīr says: "What shall I say about that (state of consciousness) on which even Brahmā and Maheś are silent? The Name of Rāma is the only way (to attain Salvation). That is the instruction of everybody (i.e., every Saint)."

Note: Brahmā (the Creator) and Maheśa or Maheśvara (Lord Śiva – the Master of Yogis) who are symbols of the greatest wisdom, are always in the "Kriyār para avasthā", the state of absolute calm. Anybody who has attained this state remains absorbed in Supreme Consciousness (Rāma). For him everything else is meaningless and futile.

Kabīr yinha yyāysā Hari jāniā, tinhakoñ tyāysā lābh
yyāyse pias no bhajāi, yab lāgi dhase na ār. ***8.***

Kabīr says that a devotee gains to the extent he has known the Lord. The thirst of a thirsty man is removed to the extent he drinks water. If he drinks water to his saturation, his thirst will be quenched completely.

Note: The man who can stay in the "Kriyār para avasthā" for a little while and has to come down again to the mundane consciousness, has not yet completed his Sādhanā. The real Saint is always absorbed in the Supreme Consciousness, in the "Kriyār para avasthā".

Kabīr Rām Nām ki lut hāy, luṭi śake so luṭ
Pheri pāche pachtāhuge, yab tan yāñihe chut. ***9.***

Kabīr says: "The Name of Rāma is there for you to take. If you do not take it, you will have to repent at the time of death".

Note: There is ample wealth (spiritual) for us in the "Kriyār para avasthā", and we can have it only through a continued practice of Kriyās.

Kabīr is duniāme āikyeya, choṛi deo tom āñyeṭ
Lenā hoy so leile, uṭhi yātu hāy pāyeṭ. ***10.***

Kabīr says: "You have come to this world only for a short while. Do not therefore be proud. And if you have to take anything, take it now; for every moment your vital breath is moving towards death."

Note: Without vanity, we must fully utilize our transitory life by practicing Kriyās.

Kabīr kuru bande tu bandegi, yo pāoye pāk didār
Āoñsar mānukh janma kā, hoy nā bārambār. ***11.***

Kabīr says: "If you want to worship God, do it now; for the human birth cannot always be had."

Note: To worship the Lord properly one should go on practicing Kriyās so long as one has physical strength.

Kabīr yohi mārag sāñi mile, tāñhi calo kari hos
Pheri pāche pachtāoge, kahe nā mānasī roṣ. ***12.***

Kabīr says: "Tread cautiously along the path which leads to Brahman. You will otherwise have to repent and suffer from anger."

Note: While practicing Kriyās, the devotee should strictly follow the instructions of his Master (Guru).

Kabīr bār bār to soñ kahuñ, śunre manuā nīc
Baṇijārāke bayel yeño, pyāyre māhi mic. ***13.***

Kabīr says: "O my low mind! Listen to what I repeatedly tell you. You are roaming uselessly like a trader's bullock (which carries the trader's goods, on its back for sale in the markets)."

Note: The human mind, attached to petty worldly gains, is like a beast of burden roaming about in bondage. The path of its emancipation lies only through the Kriyās practiced under the able guidance of a Master.

Baṇijāre ke bayel yeño, ṭāṇḍā utrā āy
Ek nahake dunā bhāyi, ek cale mūl goñāy. ***14.***

The trader's bullock becomes free when the burdens from both sides are taken off. Some of the bullocks cause double gain for the trader; some again lose even the capital.

Note: Through a practice of Kriyās all earthly attachments gradually wear off. The Prāṇa-Vāyu, which generally flows through the two gangliated cords of Sympathetic Nerves (Īṛā and Pingalā), flows through the Suṣumnā (the spinal cord) by means of the Kriyā. This means a definite gain for the spiritual life of the devotee. He makes a double gain when through 'Khecarī Mudrā' he can raise his tongue towards the 'Kûṭastha' (the two-petalled lotus in between the eye-brows: inside the body), because at this stage he can switch off his contact with the outside world at his mere wish and can therefore adjust himself with equal ease with the outside as well as the spiritual world. The greatest gain, however, is for the man who loses all earthly attachments and becomes immersed in an All-pervasive Divine Consciousness in the "Kriyār para avasthā".

Kabīr baṇijāreke bayel yeoñ, bharmat phire cauhuñ deś
Khāñṛ lahe bhūṣ khātu hāy, bin Satguru upadeś. ***15.***

Kabīr says that the trader's bullock roams about in all directions with a load of dried sugar-cane juice on its back. It is merely a carrier of the delicious food, a beast of burden. While carrying its precious load, however, the bullock is taking chaff as its own food. This is also the lot of an uninitiated man. For want of Sadguru's instructions he tastes only the chaff of this earth, leaving spiritual nourishment aside.

Note: The mind of a man who does not practice Kriyās moves restlessly from one earthly attachment to another. He is merely a bearer of the Kûṭastha within his body, without tasting its spiritual Bliss.

Kabīr Hari kā Nām le, tyaji Māyā bikh boj
Bārbār nāñhi pāi ho, mānukh janam ki moj. ***16.***

Kabīr says: "Leaving aside the poison of Māyā (mundane attachment), take the Name of Hari (the Lord); for you may not repeatedly have the advantage of a human body."

Note: Since Real Bliss can only be had in the "Kriyār para avasthā" and since this state of Consciousness can only be reached through Kriyās in the human body, the human birth is very important. So long as we have this body, therefore, we must not neglect practicing Kriyās. Lust for power, money or sexual satisfaction can never be subdued except through spiritual practices under the guidance and instructions of a Saint (Sadguru).

Kabīr jorā āye jor kiyā, piyā āpnā pahicān
Lenā hoi so leile, uṭhat hāy kharihān. ***17.***

Kabīr says: "When the breathing (here, Prāṇāyāma) in your body becomes very strong, you will come to know your Lord. Ask him anything you want. The harvest should be stored up in the granary at the proper time. (With Self-Realizaion the mind is full with spiritual harvest and has complete satisfaction)."

Note: With vigorous practice of Kriyās, the Prāṇa-Vāyu flows through the Suṣumnā (the subtle passage within the spinal cord), and gradually "Kriyār para avasthā" is attained. All earthly desires are eliminated at this stage and the devotee becomes full of Divine Bliss.

Kabīr youvan yāsi deñha tyaji, cale niśān bajāy
Śir par śvet sarāycā, diyā buṛhāpā āy. ***18.***

Kabīr says that when youth leaves the body, it goes away after hoisting the flag of grey hair. Old age now comes in.

Note: Youth is the best time for practicing Kriyās, for it is at this time that the body remains fit. Since, however, youth is transitory, we should try to make the best of it from the point of view of Kriyās.

Kabīr jorā āye jor kiyā, yoyāni dinha piṭ
Āñkhan upar ke culi, bikh bhar khāye mīṭh. ***19.***

Kabīr says: "Now that youth has made room for old age, the body is unfit to practice Kriyā with vigor. The limbs are slackened; the eyes have developed cataracts. The organs are suffering from the poisonous reactions of things formerly taken as sweets."

Note: Unless one takes initiation from a Sadguru at the young age and goes on practicing Kriyā with care, one finds it very difficult to go on with Sādhanā at the old age.

Kabīr kaṛanha lāgi bol kahe, man nehi māne hāri
Rāj berāji hot hāy, śāke to Rām sambhāri. ***20.***

Kabīr says that an old man becomes short of hearing and easily irritated. He cannot adjust himself to varied circumstances, (when something happens according to his desire, he is satisfied; otherwise he feels very much agitated). Only Rāma can save him from these troubles.

Note: Kriyā is the worship of Rāma (the Lord). If the devotee has a prolonged habit of practicing Kriyās, he can easily overcome the troubles inherent in old age.

Kabīr uñcā diśei dhau raharā, maṛhi citāoye śol
Ek Harike nām binu, yam pāṛega rol. ***21.***

Kabīr says that in old age spiritual practices seem to be too high and distant. Then again, the old man is deeply attached to his children. In these circumstances it is only the Name of Shri Hari (the Lord) which can save him. Otherwise Yāma (the god of death) will make him cry.

Note: It is very difficult to start practicing Kriyā in old age. But it is Kriyā alone which can save man from the clutches of death. Physical death is inevitable. But one who has reached "Kriyār para avasthā" is not overcome by death in the sense that he has not to be born again and again, and die. Since, therefore, Kriyā is essential for reaching the highest Consciousness, we should start practicing it in our young age when the body remains fit.

Kabīr tyajl chuṭā saharme, kasbe pari pukār
Daroyājā diyā raha, nikli geyā asoyār. **22.**

Kabīr says that the mind which is like a horse rushes out from the body which is like a city. Small areas of the city are crying. But the rider goes out.

Note: At the time of death when the Kûṭastha (the Jīvātmā) is about to leave the body riding the horse of the mind, organs of the body like the eyes, ears, hands and feet, become lifeless and inert. Since death must come, we should get ready for it by merging our Consciousness with the Divine through a long practice of Kriyās.

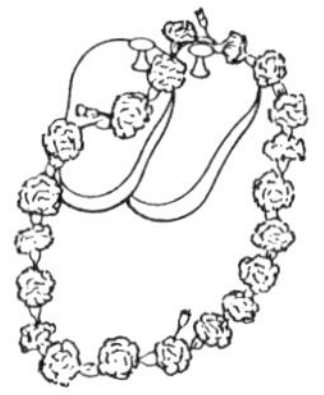

Chapter - 7

On Bhakti or Devotion

Bhakti dilāol upaji, lyāye Rāmānand
Pargaṭ kiyā Kabīrji, sāt dwīp nao khaṇd. ***1.***

Shri Rāmānanda (the Guru of Kabīr) sowed the seeds of Bhakti and Kabīr manifested it in the body having seven islands (seven principal nerve-cords) and nine doors (two eyes, two ears, two nostrils, the mouth, the penis and the anus).

Note: Kabīr, disciple of the Great Saint Rāmānanda, was inspired by his Master to worship the Paramātmā (the Supreme Self) through Kriyās in which the devotee has to close up the nine channels of the body and stop contact with the outside world for the time being and send the Prāṇa-Vāyu through all the nerve-cords in the body.

Kabīr Bhakti niśenī Mukti ki, caṛe sant sabh dhāye
Yinha Prāṇī ālas kiyā, janma gaye jahaṛāye. ***2.***

Kabīr says that Bhakti (devotion) is the symbol of Mukti (liberation from bondage). The Saints have all taken shelter in Bhakti. He who does not try to attain devotion to the Lord leads a fruitless life.

Note: Saints always remain in the "Kriyār para avasthā". But only a devoted practice of Kriyās leads one to that state of highest devotion to (and consequent identification with) the Lord.

Kabīr kāj chare nahiñ Bhakti bin, lāk kathaye yao kaye
Śabda sanehi hoy rahe, gharko pañhucey śoye. ***3.***

Kabīr says that without Bhakti no useful purpose will be served. Mere words, even millions of them, will be fruitless. The purpose of life can be fulfilled only for those who have concentrated their minds in the inner sound of Ohmkāra or have reached the Source of that sound (i.e., Sahasrāra, within the head).

Note: When due to a long and devoted practice of Kriyās the breath becomes still, the sound of Ohmkāra is heard from within. It is through a greater and greater concentration in this holy sound that the mind reaches the Sahasrāra (the thousand-petalled lotus within the head) and gets merged in Divine Consciousness. This can only be achieved by the man who has great faith in and devotion to his Guru's instructions.

Kabīr kṣet bigāre khaṇthua sabhā bigāre kur
Bhakti bigāre lālcī, yeño keśarīme dhūr. **4.**

Kabīr says that as the crops in a field are damaged by weeds, as a meeting is broken by the presence of a leper, as keśarī ('jāfrān', a fragrant spice) is wasted by its mixture with dust, so Bhakti is destroyed by Avarice.

Note: Sincere devotion to the instructions of the Sadguru is incompatible with earthly hankerings. Kriyā should be practiced with devotion irrespective of whether our desires are satisfied or not.

Kabīr trimiri gai rabi dekhte, kumti gai Gurujñān
Satya gai ek lobhte, Bhakti gai abhimān. **5.**

Kabīr says that darkness is destroyed by the Sun, evil propensity is destroyed by the wisdom imparted by the Sadguru, Truth is destroyed by Avarice, and Devotion is destroyed by egotism.

Note: Through a long practice of Kriyās the devotee sees Divine Light (the Sun) in the Kûṭastha and thus his ignorance is dispelled. Kriyā is the Grace of Shriguru and it is through Kriyā that our nature is purified. Avarice and egotism are causes of bondage from which Kriyā alone can save us.

Kabīr Bhakti bhāo bhādo nadī, sabhe cale ghaharāye
Salitā soi sarāhiye, yo jeth mās ṭhaharāye. **6.**

Kabīr says that Bhakti is like a river in the month of Bhādra (August-September, just after the rainy season in India when the rivers are full to the brim), which carries the devotee along with its strong current. He, however, who can move along with the meagre current of the month of Jyaiṣṭha (May-June, scorching Summer, when the rivers have very little water), is the best sailor.

Note: When the devotee reaches the "Kriyār para avasthā" for the first time, he is swept along the current of Divine Consciousness. But the man for whom this highest Consciousness has become easy through a long practice is not upset even in the most difficult circumstances.

Kabīr kaheñ pukri kai, kya paṇdit kyā śekh
Bhakti hetu śabde gahe, bahuri nā kāchai bhekh. ***7.***

Kabīr shouts to the Pandit (Sanskrit scholar) as well as to the Sheikh (Muslim scholar) and asks them to concentrate in the (Divine) Sound (Ohmkāra). In that case no outward show of a devotee like the sandalpaste mark (of the Vaiṣṇava, the worshipper of God in the shape of Lord Viṣṇu) or the kaupīna (the loin-cloth of the Sannyāsin) will be necsessary.

Note: Kriyāyoga, practiced sincerely, will lead the devotee to a concentrated experience of the Divine.

Kabīr kāmī krodhī lālcī, inhate Bhakti nā hoye
Bhakti kare kai śūrīyāñ, tan man lajjā khoye. ***8.***

Kabīr says that persons addicted to lust, anger and avarice, cannot attain Bhakti. Only a hero who can overcome bondage to body, mind and shame, is fit for Bhakti.

Note: Lust is that of the body. Anger and Avarice appertain to the mind. Persons with these characteristics always hanker after some concrete objects. Kriyā (worship of the Divine) is the only way which makes the devotee overcome the dirt and dross of the body and mind. The man who practices Kriyā, also gains the strength to neglect the ridicule and criticism of others and thus he overcomes the feeling of shame.

Kabīr Bhakti doar hāy śāñkra, rahl daśaye bhāy
Man airāot hoye rahā, kis bidhi payṭā yāy. ***9.***

Kabīr says that the passage to Bhakti is very subtle and it can be reached very subtly through the ten Indriyas (sense-organs). The mind is as obtuse as an elephant and therefore how can it enter into Bhakti?

Note: Bhakti is very difficult to be attained. All our sense-organs should be controlled by Kriyās and turned inwards before we can reach Bhakti in the "Kriyār para avasthā". Without Kriyās the mind becomes restless and at this state cannot be concentrated in the Divine. Thus "Bhakti" is unattainable by a restless mind which only moves on from one attachment to another.

Kabīr jñān na bedhiā, hirdayā nahiñ juṛāye
Dekhādekhi Bhakti kare, ranga nañhi ṭhāharāye. ***10.***

Kabīr says that without Realization the heart (of a devotee) cannot be satisfied. They who make a mere show of Bhakti cannot attain real satisfaction.

Note: It is only in the "Kriyār para avasthā" that Bhakti (entire devotion to God) can be attained. A mere show of Bhakti without practice of Kriyās cannot give us the Supreme Bliss which we have in the "Kriyār para avasthā".

Kabīr chemā kṣet bhal jotiye, sumiraṇ bīj jamāye
khaṇda Brahmāṇda śukhā parai, Bhakti bīj nahi yāye. ***11.***

Kabīr says: "Plow the field of forgiveness very well and sow there the seeds of concentration. The Universe may be destroyed, but Bhakti cannot be dried up".

Note: The Yogī forgives the harsh words of people from a higher consciousness. For cultivation of this higher consciousness he goes on practicing Kriyā in which the plowshare is Suṣumna, and the bullocks are Īṛā and Pingalā. The seed is concentration in the Divine or "Kriyār para avasthā" which gives him permanent Bliss. The miniature Universe is the Kûṭastha or the two-petalled plexus in between the eye-brows. A Yogī who has only reached the Kûṭastha may again come down to a lower level of consciousness, but one who stays in the "Kriyār para avasthā", in a permanent concentration in the Divine, can never have a fall.

Yeño jal pyāro machri, lobhī pyāro dām
Māt hi pyāro bālakā, Bhakti piyār Rām. ***12.***

Kabīr says that as the fish cannot live without water, as a greedy man cannot live without money, and as a child cannot live without its mother, so also Bhakti can never live without Rāma (the Lord).

Note: A person who really loves God, cannot live without concentration in the Divine. But such concentration can only be attained after a long practice of Kriyās.

Kabīr Bhaktī bhekh baṛa antarā, yaicheñ dharaṇī akāś
Bhakta yo sumirai Rām kau, bhekh jagt ki āś. ***13.***

Kabīr says that the difference between Bhakti and a mere show of it is as great as between the sky and the earth. The Bhakta (devotee) thinks only of Rāma, but the hypocrite thinks only of worldly gains.

Note: The real devotee stays in the "Kriyār para avasthā" which is an ethereal state of consciousness. Such a man is a real Yogī who is as unattached and as little upset as the sky itself. Lack of practice in the Kriyās compels the mind of man to be fettered by the bondage of earthly desires.

Kabīr par nāñ tāte hot hai, mante kiyai bhāo
Paramārath paratīt me, eba tan rahe ki yāo. ***14.***

Kabīr says: "You are mistaking an alien thing (the body with sense-organs) for Paramātmā, and doing all sorts of things according to the dictates of your mind. But when you will really have Self-Realization, you will not be anxious for your body."

Note: In the "Kriyār para avasthā", the soul becomes independent of the body and therefore, can easily neglect bodily pains and pleasures.

Kabīr yab tab Bhakti sakamatā, tab tak nihaphal seo
Kahe Kabīr ohoñ koño mile, nihamkāmī nij deo. ***15.***

Kabīr says that so long as Bhakti is mixed up with hankering after worldly gains, it is fruitless. When it is free from such hankerings, it leads to Self-Realization.

Note: Kriyā is to be practiced with devotion without worry for earthly success or failure.

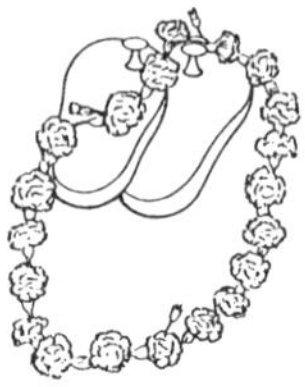

Chapter - 8

On Love

Eha to ghar hai Premkā, khālā ka ghar nāhiñ
Śiṣ utāre bhūin dhare, so paiṭe ghar māhi. ***1.***

Kabīr says that our body is the room for Love and for nothing else. He who can bend his head towards the ground can enter the zone of Love.

Note: Kriyā canalizes the Prāṇa-Vāyu from the Mūlādhāra to the Sahasrāra and again back to Mūlādhāra. The process ultimately leads us to "Kriyār para avasthā" when the mind is merged in the Divine in the Sahasrāra, and we attain Love Divine.

Kabīr śiṣ utāre bhūñi dhare, upar rākhe pāño
Dās Kabīrā eyoñ kahe, yyāysā hoyeto āo. **2.**

Kabīr says: "If you can keep your head towards the ground and your feet upwards, you will reach your destination."

Note: When, after a long practice of Kriyās, the Prāṇa-Vāyu settles down in the Sahasrāra, the Divine Energy (Kuṇḍalinī) remains in a straight line in the Suṣumnā, from head to foot, from Sahasrāra to Mūlādhāra. It is then that the Sādhaka attains Supreme Realization.

Kabīr eha to ghar hāy Premkā, mārag agam agādh
Śīs Kāṭ pālrā dhare, lāge Prem Samādh. **3.**

Kabīr says that this is the space for Love; and this is the way to the inaccessible. If the scales are made equal by cutting the head off, the Ecstasy of Love Divine will be produced.

Note: It is the Sahasrāra which is the seat for Love Divine and the "Kriyār para avasthā" is the real state of this Love. This state of Consciousness, this utmost repose and tranquillity, however, is completely inaccessible to anybody whose mind is restless. Īṛā and Pingalā have been compared to the two sides of a scale. But when the string joining these two sides is cut off, the sides become balanced. The Prāṇa-Vāyu moving into the Suṣumnā and reaching the head is like cutting off the scales of Īṛā and Pingalā.

Kabīr Prem Bhaktikā ghaṛā, uñcā bahutak māth
Śīṣ kāṭ pagutar dhare, tab pañouchegā hāt. **4.**

Kabīr says that the pitcher of Love Divine is higher even than the head. It cannot be touched by hand unless the head is held beneath the feet.

Note: The Kriyā should be practiced with Love. But even then it is very difficult to reach the head. It is only when the Prāṇa-Vāyu settles within the head in the "Kriyār-para avasthā", that there is an equal pressure from head to foot and the devotee reaches the state of utter tranquillity and perfection of the Love Divine.

Kabīr Prem na bāri upaje, Prem na hāṭ bikāy
Binā Premkā mānoyā, bāndhā Yampur yāy. **5.**

Kabīr says that Love does not come out of water; Love is not sold in the market. A man without Love is led in fetters into the land of Death.

Note: Love Divine can only be attained in the "Kriyār para avasthā" when the devotee feels that everything in this Universe is Brahman. It cannot grow merely by physical penance which sucks the juice of the body. It cannot also be gained through a business mentality by bargaining with the Lord. So long as earthly desires are predominant, there cannot be liberation for the soul. And the soul in bondage can never taste the ecstacy of Love Divine.

Kabīr śīṣ utāran na kāhā, dinho bhāo batāye
Tino lok kā śīṣ hāy jore utārā yāye. **6.**

Kabīr says: "Actually I have not spoken of the cutting off of the head. By that I wanted to mean a particular state of spiritual consciousness. There are heads for all three worlds and they can be pulled down by force."

Note: By severance of the head Kabīr has meant the "Kriyār para avasthā". By the three worlds Kabīr has meant the Heaven, the Earth and the Nether World corresponding respectively to the head, the heart and the feet. When the Prāṇa-Vāyu moves with force from head to foot, the plexuses in all three places are joined as it were in One Divine consciousness. This is the significance of the cutting off of the heads or crests in the different nerve-centres of the body.

Kabīr Prem piyālā so piye, yo śīṣ dacctiṇā dey
Lobhi śīṣ nā de śake, nām Premkā ley. ***7.***

Kabīr says that a man who has given his head to his Master as a tribute drinks the cup of nectar. Greedy persons cannot offer their heads in a like manner, because their love is not genuine.

Note: Offering the head to Shriguru means the state of Samādhi, because in that state of consciousness there is no separate existence of the limited consciousness of man. 'Head' is generally taken as the seat of intellect and therefore, the devotee in the "Kriyār para avasthā", by surrendering his separate will, is said to have offered his head to his Master.

Kabīr śīṣ kāṭ paṣangā kiyā, jīu surāhī bharilīn
yehi bhāve so āile, Prem āmi kahi din. ***8.***

Kabīr says: "By cutting the head and breaking stones, the human self (Jīvātmā) has filled the pitcher of his body with Divine Love. Come, anybody who wishes to do so. This Love is unfathomable. This is the opinion of my humble self."

Note: When the Prāṇa-Vāyu, after passing through the lower centres, reaches the Sahasrāra, the Love Divine is achieved. But this is a highly difficult process which has been compared to the breaking of stones. However, this is possible through Kriyās, with the Grace of the Sadguru. Love, therefore, is achieved only in "Kriyār para avasthā".

Kabīr Prem piyālā bhari piyā, rāci rahā Gurujñān
Diyā nāgrā śabdakā, lāl khāṛe maidān. ***9.***

Kabīr says: "Drink the cup full of the nectar of Divine Love. Then you will be able to comprehend all the activities of Shriguru. You will hear 'Ohmkāra' like the beating of drums. You will then reach the field of Brahman, the most precious jewel to be sought for."

Note: If we go on practicing Kriyās we gradually become able to comprehend the words and activities of the Sadguru and reach the highest spiritual Consciousness.

Kabīr chin paṛe chin utare, so to Prem na hoy
Āṭ pahar lāgā rahe, Prem kahāoye soy. ***10.***

Kabīr says that the devotion which comes and goes cannot be called Love. Love is constant and is a companion for twenty-four hours.

Note: One who constantly remains in Divine consciousness can be said to have attained Love. This highest state of ecstasy and intoxication can only be reached in the "Kriyār para avasthā".

Kabīr āyā Prem kāñhā geyā, dekhāyā sab koy
Pal roye pal mo hāñse, so to Prem nā hoy. ***11.***

Kabīr says: "Love actually came. Where has it gone now? Everybody saw the man (who was temporarily under the intoxication of Love Divine) laughing at one moment and crying in the next. But that, too, cannot be called Love."

Note: Anybody who practices the Kriyā sincerely, reaches the "Kriyār para avasthā" sometimes. But unless that state of consciousness becomes stable and permanent, it cannot be called Love Divine in the real sense of the term.

Prem prem sabhiñ kahe, Prem nā cinhe koy
Yoñhi ghaṭ Prem-piñjar base, Prem kahāoye soy. ***12.***

Kabīr says that everybody talks about Love, but none (i.e., very few) knows or understands it. He alone can talk of Love whose head has become a cage for Love Divine.

Note: Unless one has reached the "Kriyār para avasthā", one cannot comprehend the true nature of constant communion with the Divine.

Kabīr Prem na cinhiyā cākhi no kinho soyādey
Śune gharkā pāhunā, yeño āoye teoñ yāy. ***13.***

Kabīr says: "I have not yet been able to comprehend or taste Love. It came, just like a guest to an uninhabited house, and went away."

Note: The ordinary sense of the above lines expresses Kabīr's modesty. Of course Kabīr has known Love Divine. But the lines may also be taken in a deeper spiritual sense. The 'Kriyār para avasthā' is a state of complete identification with God. Since there is no separate existence of the devotee, how can there be any recognition of something separate from himself? It is he who is Love Divine.

Kabīr Prem piyāre lāl so, man mo kinho bhāo
Sat Guruke Pratāp te, bhālā banā hāy dāño. ***14.***

Kabīr says that Love is his dearest. Through the influence of the Sadguru his mind has established contact with this dearest. And this has actually turned to be the most profitable deal for him.

Kabīr eha tan jvāroñ masi karoñ, likho Rām ko Nām
Likhnī karo karak ki, likhi likhi paṭhāo Rām. ***15.***

Kabīr says: "Prepare the ink after burning your body and write the Name of Rāma with that. Make your mind the pen of troubles and send the writing."

Note: The pen symbolizes 'Kriyā'. The trouble taken by the devotee in practicing Kriyās leads the mind gradually to 'Kriyār para avasthā" where the mind becomes as colorless as ashes, because there is no separate existence for it. Practicing Kriyās has been described as burning the body. Kriyā destroys all the dirt and dross of the human body and mind.

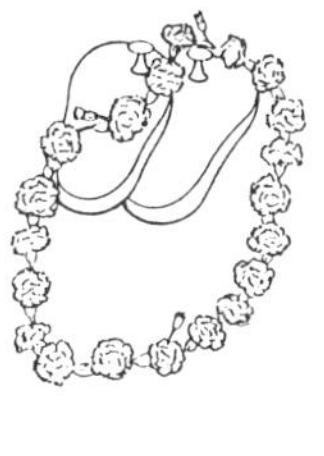

Chapter - 9

On the Grief of Separation

Kabīr pīr pirāṇī birha ki, āor nā kachu so hāye
Yāysi pīr hāy birha ki, rahi kaleje chāye. ***1.***

Kabīr says that his heart has been overwhelmed with the pain of separation from the Divine and therefore nothing can make him cheerful.

Note: Whenever we lose contact with the Divine, after having attained it for once, we are thrown into a state of agony till we reach "Kriyār para avasthā" again. Such agony, however, can only come to a man who constantly practices Kriyā to reach the highest state of consciousness permanently.

Kabīr coṭ santāoye birha ki, sab tan jhanjharā hoye
Mar nihārā jānchi, ki yiskā lāgi hoye. **2.**

Kabīr says that due to the intensity of the pain of separation the entire body has been full of pores (i.e., consumed). Only he who has suffered this pain knows how agonizing it is.

Note: If we fetch water in a pitcher having countless pores, all the water comes out leaving nothing within the pitcher. So also the devotee suffering separation from the Divine becomes utterly careless of his body which seems to him like a vacant casket containing nothing.

Kabīr biraha bhajangam tan dacheo, mantra na lāge koy
Rām biyogī nā jīñye, jīñye to bāyura hoy. ***3.***

Kabīr says: "The serpent of Separation bites the human body. No charm or sacred chant can effectively neutralize the poison of this snake. A man suffering the agony of separation from Rāma (the Divine) cannot live, or if he lives at all, he lives like a mad man (mad with the yearning of a union with the Divine)."

Note: After having reached the Transcendent state of Consciousness we may again be thrown back into earthly life. This is a state of intense pain which is mitigated only when, after a prolonged practice of Kriyās, our consciousness settles forever in the "Kriyār para avasthā", never to fall again. It is this state of permanent Bliss which is called "Brāhmī Sthiti" (staying in Brahman or the Lord) in the *Gītā*. This Bliss, however, comes and goes before the devotee is permanently settled in it.

Kabīr birha bhujangam paiṭhike, kiyā kaleje ghāo
Birhiṇī ang an moṛai, yo bhāoye to khāo. ***4.***

Kabīr says that the serpent of separation has made the heart its seat and has eaten into its vitals; but the lady (i.e., the devotee who is hankering after a union with the Divine) goes on suffering the pain without any movement of her limbs. "Now eat what thou wilt", says Kabīr .

Note: After tasting the Divine Bliss through Kriyās the devotee (likened to a female yearning after union with her beloved) cannot apply his mind to material possessions. This is what is meant by the expression that he does not move his limbs. In such a state of consciousness his only food would be to taste the nectar of Divine Consciousness.

Kabīr rag rag baje rabāb tan, biraha santāye nit
Aor na koe śunsi, Sāñ: śune ki cit. ***5.***

Kabīr says that the musical sound (Ohmkāra) is ringing within every vein in the body; but due to the agony of separation the devotee cannot listen to it. It is only the Lord who is hearing this sound.

Note: Although the Ohmkāra is ringing all the time within our bodies, we are not able to hear it. It is only the man who has fixed his mind in the Supreme Being who can hear Ohmkāra. But for that, practice of Kriyā is essential.

Kabīr biraha yo āyo daraś ko, Kaṛuā lāgā kām
Kāyā lāgi kāl hoye, miṭhā lāgā Rām. ***6.***

Kabīr says that when Separation found that this body was the root of all evil, it took all desires as evil. Only the Name of Rāma seemed to be sweet. Everything else became meaningless.

Note: Once the devotee feels the Divine in the Kûṭastha, he loses attachment to everything except the Kriyās which would lead him again to his union with the Lord.

Kabīr iha tan ko dīyalā karo, bāti melo jīu
Lohu sico tel kari, tab mukh dekha piu. ***7.***

Kabīr says: "Make your body the lamp, make Jīvātmā (the human consciousness) the wick, and use the blood within you veins as the oil. Then alone you will be able to see the Face of your Beloved (viz., the Divine)."

Note: The body becomes a lamp when through a long practice of Kriyās the devotee sees Divine Light all the time. To practice Kriyā with vigor is to set the wick of the lamp in order and oil it in the proper manner. The result of all this is a union with the Divine in the "Kriyār para avasthā".

Kabīr biraha binā tan śunya hāy, biraha hāy Sultān
Yā ghaṭ biraha na sañcāre, so ghaṭ jānu maśān. ***8.***

Kabīr says that without the feeling of separation the body has become empty. Separation exerts its influence like a king. The pitcher (i.e., the human body) in which 'separation' has not found its place is like a burial ground, for it denotes a lack of love for the Divine.

Note: A man who has never experienced Divine Love cannot feel separation. And the way to achieve Love Divine is the Kriyā. The man practicing Kriyā proceeds alternately through union with and separation from the Divine, till he permanently settles in the Transcendent Consciousness where there is absolute union with the Supreme.

Kabīr biraha Rām pāṭhāiyāñ, Sādhunke parmodh
Ya ghaṭ tālā meli hāy, tāko lay kari sodh. ***9.***

Kabīr says that Rāma (the Lord) Himself has sent 'separation' in order to increase the intensity of Love of the virtuous. A man who has kept the lock of his heart open, achieves Samādhi in its purest form (i.e., achieves complete absorption in the Divine).

Note: The pang of separation is only in order to intensify the Love. The man who has become so much a lover of the Lord that he can attain Samādhi at the mere wish, is the most pure. His heart remains always open to receive the Grace Divine.

Kabīr āñkhṛiāñ Prem ki chuñiyā, yin jāne dukhṛia
Rām sanehi kāraṇe, roye roye rataṛiā. ***10.***

Kabīr says that the man who suffers the grief of separation waits with thirsty eyes for Divine Love. He spends the whole night weeping for union with Rāma.

Note: One who has sufficiently advanced in Kriyās, yearns after a complete merger with the Divine in the "Kriyār para avasthā."

Kabīr soi āhe su svajanā, soi āhe lokṛiāñ
Yo locan Iohu cūye, tab hiñ janiho taṛiā. ***11.***

Kabīr says that he is good whose eyes shed tears; but he whose eyes shed blood (i.e., are always red) is very near to achieving Samādhi.

Note: Tears for the Divine denote an advanced stage in the Kriyās; but blood-red eyes for one who practices Kriyā signify that he is about to settle in the "Kriyār para avasthā".

Kabīr hamsa nādari karu, ro-onā soñ karu cit
Bin roye ko pāiyā Prem piyāre mit. ***12.***

Kabīr says: "Make your Jīvātmā (i.e., yourself) the Divine Sound of Ohmkāra, i.e., make it crying for God; for without cries and lamentations who has ever been united with his beloved?"

Note: A devoted practice of Kriyās is the cry of the devotee's soul for being united with the Paramātmā in the "Kriyār para avasthā".

Kabīr so to dunkha na bisare, ro-ot balghaṭi yāye
Man hi māha bisur nā, yoñ kāṭh-hiñ ghuṇ khāye. ***13***.

Kabīr says that he cannot forget the grief (of separation). Due to much crying and lamentation his physical strength has diminished and he has also forgotten all that was there in his mind. He has therefore become like a piece of worm-eaten wood, having his inner strength sapped by grief.

Note: So long as the devotee cannot settle himself in the "Kriyār para avasthā", he has to suffer from a terrible restlessness.

Kabīr kiñṛe kāṭh yo khāiyā khaya kinahu na diṭh
So ti ughāri yo dekhiye, bhitar jāmā ciṭh. ***14.***

Kabīr says that when worms eat up a piece of wood, nobody is aware of its decay from the outside. But when somebody tries to take it up, he alone realizes that there is nothing inside but dust.

Note: The grief of the lover of God due to lack of identification with the Divine cannot always be guessed from the outside. It reveals itself only to a careful observer who himself practices Kriyā.

Kabīr ciṭh yo jāma cūṇkā, birahā baurā khay
Bisari gayā yo svajanā, bedan kāhu no law. ***15.***

Kabīr says that the devotee turns mad with Love for the Divine and feeds on the decay of his own body. But the pain of the Lord Himself is not realized by anybody.

Note: So long as "Kriyār para avasthā" does not become easy for the devotee, the grief of separation remains intense.

Kabīr hāñse piyā nahi pāiye, yinha pāyā tinha roy
Hāñsi khel yo piyā mile, to kon dohāginī hoyā. ***16.***

Kabīr says that we cannot be united with the Dearest Lord through laughter and frivolity. Everybody who has been so united had to weep for Him. If one could reach the Lord through frivolity, who, then, would become a widow?

Note: A man who has settled in the Kûṭastha can be compared to a woman having her husband alive. Such a woman has the mark of vermilion on her forehead in between the eye-brows. The devotee whose gaze has always been fixed on the two-petalled lotus can therefore be taken as one united with his beloved Lord. But the devotee who has experienced the Light Divine in the Kûṭastha but cannot get it at the mere wish is one suffering separation from the Lord. Such a man can be compared to a widow who had experienced the bliss of union with her husband, but cannot get it now. He has to go on practicing Kriyā for achieving permanent union.

Kabīr hāñsi khel yo piyā mile, to kon sahe khursān
Kām Krodh tṛṣṇā tyaje, tāhi mile Bhagvan. ***17.***

Kabīr says: "If frivolous merry-makings would lead us to God, who would practice Sādhanā as difficult as moving on a razor's edge? It is only when one conquers lust, anger and avarice that one can hope to reach the Divine."

Note: To keep the mind moving through the subtle passage of the Suṣumnā is as difficult as to move along a razor's edge. It can only be done through a constant practice of Kriyās. It is through such practice that the lower consciousness of man is gradually merged in the Supreme Consciousness. At this stage, since there is no separate existence of the human consciousness of the devotee, who will indulge in lust, anger or avarice?

Kabīr hāus kare Hari milan ki, āo sukh cāhe ang
Pīṛ sahe binu paduminī, putan let uchang. ***18.***

Kabīr says: "To want God and physical comfort at the same time is to be like a woman who wants a child but does not like to bear the labor pain."

Note: For God-Realization one must take the trouble of practicing Kriyās.

Kabīr dekhat dekhat din gayā, niśabhi dekhat yahiñ
Birahiṇī piyā pāoya nahi, jīoyat rase man māhi. ***19.***

Kabīr says that days and nights pass by, and yet the lady (Jīvātmā) remains separated from her husband (Paramātmā, the Lord) and is therefore grieved in her heart.

Note: If we do not practice Kriyās due to idleness, we have to repent for lack of Self-Realization.

Kabıī ki birahiṇīkoñ mīc de, ki āpuhi dekhlāye
Āṭ prahar kā dājh nā, moñte sāhā na yāye. ***20.***

Kabīr says: "Ask the lady (the devotee who suffers separation from the Divine) to realize for herself, because otherwise her lamentations are intolerable".

Note: The way to be united with the Divine (i.e., to have Self-Realization) is the Kriyā. This alone can ultimately banish the grief of separation by leading the devotee to the Transcendent state of Consciousness ("Kriyār para avasthā").

Kabıī birahiṇī thī to kyā bhayā, jvarin piyā ko lār
Rahure mugudha gahe lari, birahā lajo mār. ***21.***

Kabīr says: "What could be done if the Jīvātmā (human consciousness) had to suffer separation? Since she could not identify herself with the Lord and was going along the prohibited path without any feeling of shame, let her suffer like that."

Note: So long as "Kriyār para avasthā" is not attained, perfect peace and tranquillity are misnomers.

Kabīr ho-o biraha ki lakṙi samujhi samujhi ghughūāy
Duhkha so tabahiñ bāñci ho, yab sakalo jvari yāy. ***22.***

Kabīr says that the fuel of separation burns very slowly. It is only when the burning is complete, the devotee attains relief from all grief.

Note: After intense practice of Kriyās come the "Kriyār para avasthā," when the Jīvātmā relishes the Bliss of union with the Paramātmā.

Kabīr biraha agini tan mo lāgi, gaye nayan jal śukhi
Āb hute bujhe nahi, doy hāt kar kuki. ***23.***

Kabīr says that the fire of separation has affected the whole body and dried up tears. Even if one tries to quench that fire by pouring water with both hands, the fire goes on increasing.

Note: The pang of separation from the Divinie cannot be mitigated by any external appliances. It can only be quenched in the "Kriyār para avasthā" which again can be achieved after a long practice of Kriyās.

Kabīr tan man e jvalā, biraha agini śogī
Mrtak pīṛ na jānai, jāne giyo āgi. ***24.***

Kabīr says that separation from the Divine burns down the body and mind of the devotee without his knowledge, just as a dead man cannot feel any pain.

Note: To reach the "Kriyār para avasthā" is a kind of death for the devotee's physical consciousness. When he reaches the Bliss, he is another man as it were.

Kabīr Prem binā dhīraj nahi, biraha binā bairag
Nām binā yāoye nahi, man man sāko dāg. ***25.***

Kabīr says that without Love no patience can be achieved; without the grief of separation there cannot be non-attachment; without the Holy Name the impurities of the mind cannot be blotted out.

Note: Love makes one's mind concentrated on the beloved and so the lover becomes steady and patient. Again, it is the grief of separation which increases the yearning of the lover for union with his beloved, and naturally he becomes indifferent and non-attached to everything else besides his object of affection. Such concentration, when applied in regard to the Divine; makes man indifferent to all earthly joys and sorrows and leads him gradually to a perfect union with the Lord in the "Kriyār para avasthā". Kriyā is the Holy Name which gradually removes the impurities of the mind of man till he becomes perfectly pure in the "Kriyār para avasthā".

Kabīr biraha kayoṇḍal bhari liyā, bairāgī doye nayan
Pāyā daraṣ madhukarī, chaki rahe rasanā bayan. ***26.***

Kabīr says that the eyes which were so long dry due to separation from the Divine have now (in the state of union) been filled with the water of non-attachment. Now that the devotee tastes the honey-sweet Brahman, his tongue and mouth are full of the nectar of Bliss.

Note: When in the "Kriyār para avasthā" the devotee feels the presence of the Lord in everything and everywhere, he has no more any earthly wish. He becomes more than satisfied by tasting the nectar-like juice emitted from the Sahasrāra.

Kabīr nayan hamāre bāore, chin chin loṭe tujh
Nā tu mile na mai sukhī yāyse bedan mujh. ***27.***

Kabīr says: "My mad eyes (due to separation) run hither and thither. They cannot be satisfied without having something and yet cannot stop. Such is my torment."

Note: When the consciousness is lifted high due to Kriyās intermittent glimpses of the Divine make us all the more restless to have the "Kriyār para avasthā" once for all.

Kabīr phāri paṭorā dhvajā karoñ, kām lañ pahirāye
Yohi yohi bhek piyā mile, soi soi bhek banāye. ***28.***

Kabīr says: "Make your head-dress by tearing silk-cloth into pieces. Wear blankets. Adopt any insignia that is necessary for proceeding along the path of the Divine."

Note: Silk cloth stands for pride of wealth. Tearing silk cloth denotes breaking off this pride. This can only be done by one whose 'Prāṇa-Vāyu' has settled in the Sahasrāra within the head, i.e., one who has reached 'Kriyār para avasthā'. Wearing a blanket symbolizes adoption of a humble man's dress. Humility makes it easier to reach the Divine. Pride of anything takes our minds away from Him.

Kabīr parbat parbat myāy phira, nayan gañoyāye roye
So buṭī pāoye nahīñ, yāte sarjīban hoye. ***29.***

Kabīr says: "I have roamed about from mountain to mountain and have lost my eyes through weeping; Yet I could not have that medicinal root by which I could conquer death".

Note: Due to restlessness of mind we move here and there and everywhere in search of a holy man, with the hope of lasting Divine Bliss. But our search remains fruitless till at last we receive the Sadguru who initiates us with the Kriyā which alone can lead us to the Deathless Reality.

Biraha tej tan mor rahāy, ang sabhe akulāy
Ghaṭ śūno jīuo piu omo, maut dhuñṛi phir yāy. ***30.***

Kabīr says: "Separation has had its effects on my body, and my limbs have almost been numbed. The pitcher of the body has almost become empty. Although the Jīvātmā is still within the body, he is united with the Lord. Hence, Death goes back without finding the Jīvātmā in the body."

Note: After realizing his identity with the Divine the devotee understands that his real Self is not the body, but the Paramātmā. Is the body, then, non-existent? No, the body is there; but since the Consciousness has reached Brahman, the devotee is no more attached to his bodily pleasure or pain.

Kabīr berā pāyā sarapkā, bhaosāgar ke māhi
Yab chāre tao buṛi maro, gañho to ḍache bāñhi. ***31.***

Kabīr says: "I have got a snake-boat in order to cross the Ocean of worldliness. If I do not accept its help, I shall be drowned. If, on the other hand, I catch hold of it, it will bite my hand."

Note: The Divine Energy within the body is called the 'Kuṇḍalinī' and is likened to a serpent. This Energy lies latent in the Mūlādhāra and is awakened through Kriyās received from a Sadguru. The Energy then runs along the Suṣumnā (the very subtle passage within the spinal cord) through the different plexuses and ultimately reaches the Sahasrāra in the "Kriyār para avasthā". Hence it is the Kuṇḍalinī which makes us overcome the earthly Consciousness and reach the Divine. But at the same time the devotee has to mould himself completely anew in order to reach the Life Divine.

Kabīr nayan hamāre bichohīyā rahore śamkha ma jhur
Deoal deoal māy phiro, deocha ugā nahi sur. ***32.***

Kabīr says: "My eyes still suffer from separation, because they are unable to see now what they saw for once. I have also moved from one deity to another, but unfortunately, the night of my grief has not yet ended, and the Sun has not yet been revealed to me."

Note: The devotee has seen the Sun-like effulgence of the Ātmā in the Kûṭastha, but now he can no more recapture it. He has to go on practicing Kriyās before he can see the Divine Radiance whenever he wishes.

Kabīr galo tumhāre Nām par, yoñ āṭe me loṇ
Yyāysā birāhā meli ho nit duhkh pāoye kon. ***33.***

Kabīr says: "My mind melts in Thy (God's) Name, just as salt is merged in flour. Who will suffer constant grief if he is united with the Divine after experiencing separation?"

Note: Kriyā leads to "Kriyā para avasthā", where our human consciousness is merged in the Divine, and all other sufferings end.

Kabīr sukhīyā sabh samsār hāy, khāoye śo-oye nit
Duhkhīa Dās Kabīr hāy, jāge sumire cit. ***34.***

Kabīr says: "Everybody in his world seems to be happy, for everybody is taking food and sleeping without worry. I alone am unhappy, for I have always to keep myself wide awake to think of God, lest I forget Him."

Note: Most people in this world are indifferent to anything but creature-comforts. The devotee, however, should shake off idleness in order to practice Kriyā which alone would ultimately lead man to Perfect Bliss.

Kabīr biraha jvālāi myāy jvaloñ, jvalti jvalahar yāyo
Mahi dekhat jvalahar jvare, so to kāñhāñ bujhāyo. ***35.***

Kabīr says: "I have been burnt up in the fire of Separation. He who was the cause of my burning has also been burnt up, i.e., has been identified with His devotee. Now the sensation of burning, too, is nowhere to be found."

Note: The feeling of separation from the Divine ends when the devotee settles permanently in the "Kriyār para avasthā".

Kabīr biraha jvālāi myāy jvaloñ, mujhe biraha ka duhkha
Chāhan bayṭhat ḍarpati, mati jvari yāoye rukh. ***36.***

Kabīr says that he was burnt in the fire of separation and depressed in grief. There was no happiness for him. He was afraid even to sit under a shade, lest the shade itself might be burnt due to his intense grief of separation.

Note: The devotee who has once felt the Divine due to the Grace of the Sadguru, hankers after a constant union in the "Kriyār para avasthā". So long as he cannot have it, he has to suffer intense agony.

Kabīr birahiṇī jvalti dekh kay, Sāñi āye dhāy
Prem bundte sici kay, tan me layi milāy. ***37.***

Kabīr says that seeing His beloved (the devotee who has been compared to a lady mad with love for the Divine) burning, the Lord Himself came running. He sprinkled upon her drops of His own Love and absorbed her within Himself.

Note: Prolonged practice of Kriyās makes the devotee fix his gaze at the central point in the Kûṭastha and leads him to the Transcendent state of Consciousness where he is ultimately united with the Divine.

Kabīr myāy birahiṇī ke pīṃe, dāg na diyā yāy
Mās gali gali cūñi paṛā, myāy yo rahi gale lāy. ***38.***

Kabīr says that the Lord sympathized with the grief of the beloved, but he found no space in her body to put His own mark, for the flesh had already melted away. The Lord therefore clasped her by the throat.

Note: When the grief of separation is over, and the devotee becomes united for ever with the Kûṭastha, he becomes utterly indifferent to his physical life. So long he had to suffer intense pain of separation which had transformed his body into skin and bones. Now, that pain is over, and his consciousness has triumphantly come out of the physical plane of reality.

Kabīr cāri pāoke palang śo coli lāyo āgi
Yā kāraṇ e tāttākiā, soi nā gale lāgi. ***39.***

Kabīr says that he has laid himself on a cot, and his body had started burning. But still he cannot clasp the throat of Him for whom he has taken so much trouble.

Note: The devotee keeps his body straight while practicing Kriyās and the Fire of Divine Consciousness runs through his spine, and yet it is a long way to get identified with the Lord.

Kabīr koye kara kaṭṭoriā, muṭhi kara gahi hāṛ
Yich piñjare birahā base, māsu kāñhāñre dāṛ. ***40.***

Kabīr says that he has kept the well within his hand just like a small pot, for it is difficult for him to raise water from the well, as his body has become so weak due to separation that it is nothing but skin and bones.

Note: Constant practice of Kriyās has made the body emaciated, but it has placed the well of wisdom within the reach of the devotee.

Kabīr rakt māsu sabh bhachi gaye, neku na kin ho kāṇ
Ār birahā kukur bhaye, lāge hāṛ chabān. ***41.***

Kabīr says that flesh and blood have almost evaporated from his body. His ears, too, are no more in order, for he cannot hear any call. Separation, like a dog, has been eating into his bones.

Note: Prolonged practice of Kriyās turns the physical senses inward and the devotee becomes full of Divine Consciousness to his very bones.

Kabīr birahā bhayā bichāonā, oṛhaṇ bipati biyog
Duhkha śir hāne pāoñte, kon banā samyog. ***42.***

Kabīr says: "Separation has become my bed; separation has become my wrapper: separation is troubling me from head to foot. I find separation everywhere. Where, then, is union?"

Note: So long as the devotee cannot reach the state of identification with the Divine, he has to suffer intense pain.

Kabīr kon jagāoye Brahmako, kon jagāoye jīu
Kon jāgāoye surati ko, kon milāoye piu. ***43.***

Kabīr asks: "Who will awaken the Supreme? Who will rouse the Consciousness in man? Who will create the passion for union with the Divine? Who, again, will effect the union?"

Note: It is Kriyā alone which awakens the Divine Consciousness in man and leads him ultimately to a Supreme identification with God in the "Kriyār para avasthā".

Kabīr birahā jāgāoye Brahmako, Brahma jāgāoye jīu
Jīu jāgāoye surati ko, surati milāoye piu. ***44.***

Kabīr says: "It is separation which will awaken the Brahman and it is Brahman again who will rouse the human self. The human Consciousness will rouse a passionate hankering after God, and it is this hankering again which will lead to the ultimate union with the Lord."

Note: In the search for rest and peace for the human soul, Kriyā is all-important. It is Kriyā which cultivates a hankering after the Supreme Bliss which can be had only in the "Kriyār para avasthā".

Kabīr myāy tomko ḍhuṇte phiroñ, tom kāhe nā miliā Ram
Hirdayā māhi uṭhi milo, eha sakal tomāro kām. ***45.***

Kabīr says: "I have all along been searching for you, O Lord! Why do You not come? Come to my heart and make me united with Yourself. All this can after all be done by You alone."

Note: It is after all through Divine Grace that we can have our contact with the Sadguru and have Kriyā. The Grace of God and the Guru is therefore at the root of our struggle for liberation.

Kabīr biraha jāgāiyā, pari ḍhaḍhoñre chār
Myāy koi koyālā ubre, jvāro duji bār. ***46.***

Kabīr says that the fire of separation has burnt everything else. Only the coal of ego remains. Let that, too, be burnt now.

Note: The Lord grants a vision to the devotee and then becomes invisible. The devotee goes on practicing Kriyā in order to see Him again and gradually becomes purified of all his dirt and dross. But even at a very high stage of the Kriyā his separate Consciousness remains. When that, too, goes in the "Kriyār para avasthā", he becomes completely identified with God.

Kabīr tan man yauvan jvārike, bhasam yo kariyā deha
Kahahiñ Kabīr eha birahiṇī, uṭhike ṭaṭo hāy kheha. ***47.***

Kabīr says that the lady suffering from separation (i.e., the devotee) has burnt her body, mind and youth to ashes. But now she wants to get to the root of this burning.

Note: The mind of the devotee who practices Kriyā for a long time tastes nothing but Brahman and therefore all his physical senses are dead as it were to the outside world. With deep concentration he now tries to reach the Transcendent state of Consciousness.

Kabīr birahā so to haṭi rahe, manuā merā sujān
Hāṛ mās nakh kṣāt hāy, jīyate kare maśān. ***48.***

Kabīr says that separation has eaten into his vitals – flesh and bones and nails; it has made the mind and Jīvātmā (human Consciousness) as bleak as a burial ground.

Note: The intense yearning to get identified with the Lord (i.e., to have Self-Realization) makes one a **Jīvanmukta** (one who has achieved complete liberation from bondage while still in his human body). This, however, can be achieved only through a continued practice of Kriyās. But once it is achieved, the liberated man is, in a sense, dead to the work-a-day world; because his Consciousness rests on the highest plane of Reality from which everything on the mundane plane seems to be mere child's play.

Kabīr so din kyāysā hoyegā, Rām ghahige bāñhi
Āpna kari baiṭhāosi, caraṇ kañol ki chāhi. ***49.***

Kabīr asks: "When will the day dawn upon me on which Lord Rāma will take me by the hand, make me His own and seat me at the shelter of His feet?"

Note: The steadiness of breath gained through the practice of Kriyās is symbolized by the Lord Himself taking the devotee by the hand. This gradually leads him to the concentration in the Ājñā Cakra when he can have a complete surrender to the Divine Will and the consequent sense of Bliss.

Kabīr ank bhari bhari bheṭiyā, man nahi bādhe dhīr
Kahe Kabīr te ko mile, yab lagi hoye śarīr. ***50.***

Kabīr says that he sees the Lord on his lap, but the mind still remains restless. When his mind, too, will be united with the Divine, he will really have Him.

Note: Through the Kriyās the devotee might sometimes have glimpses of the Divine. But it is only when the mind loses its separate identity completely in the Divine, i.e., when the Sādhaka reaches the "Kriyār para avasthā", that the consummation of spiritual life is reached.

Kabīr jīu bilambā piucho, alakṣ lakṣa nahi yāy
Govinda mile na jhal bujhay, rahe bujhāi bujhāy. ***51.***

Kabīr says that the individual loses his consciousness in the Divine and becomes invisible like the Brahman. Whenever he reaches the Lord, the fire of separation is extinguished. Before that, the mind has to be solaced from time to time.

Note: The "Kriyār para avasthā" is a state of consciousness where there is no separation between man and God. Who, then, will be the seer and who the sight? It is in this sense that the devotee becomes non-existent and therefore invisible; because he is left with no identity separate from the Divine. So long as the "Kriyār para avasthā" is not reached, the dissatisfaction cannot be removed from the mind of the devotee. During this period it is Kriyā alone which gives the mind some solace.

Kabīr lakṛi jari koylā bheyi, mo man ajahu āgi
Biraha ki yodi lakṛi jarai, sulāgi sulāgi. **52.**

Kabīr says that the mind, burning like logs of wood, has been transformed to coal as it were. But the burning has been slow, because the logs were wet.

Note: The mind, so long as it does not reach the highest state of consciousness, cannot become perfectly pure, i.e., free from the bondage of earthly attachments. In such an imperfect state it has been compared to wet logs of wood which take a long time to be consumed by the Fire of the Divine.

Kabīr niśu din dājhai birahiṇī, antar gata ki lāye
Dās kabīrā ko bujhai, Satguru gaye lāgāye. **53.**

Kabīr says that the Sadguru has lighted the fire of separation in him and he has been suffering day and night from the burns, for the cause of this burning has gone far away from him. None excepting the sufferer can realize the intensity of this pain.

Note: The Sadguru, after initiating the disciple into Kriyā, grants him an experience of the Divine. Such experience, however, can only be regained after a long and devoted practice of Kriyās. In the meantime the Sādhaka has to suffer from intense yearning after union with the Divine.

Kabīr śuṣat baṛa rukhṛā, myāy jan latṛiā
Tere Nām bilāmiā, yyoñ jal machṛiā. **54.**

Kabīr says that separation has made him very dry, and yet he, like a creeper, remains intertwined with God's Name, just like a fish living in water.

Note: Kriyā gradually eliminates the restlessness of the human mind till at last the mind itself is merged in Supreme Consciousness in the "Kriyār para avasthā".

Kabīr yo jan birahī Nāmke, jhine pajar tāsu
Nayan na āoye nidri, ang na jāmai māsu. **55.**

Kabīr says that the man who suffers the pain of separation from the Divine all the time, has his rib-bones exposed due to emaciation. He can neither sleep nor put on flesh on his body.

Note: The man who practices Kriyā, but has not yet reached the "Kriyār para avasthā", has to suffer from an intense yearning after union with the Divine.

Kabīr yo jan birahī Nāmke, tinha ki gati bhaiyeha
Dehī soñ udim kare, sumiraṇ kare bideha. ***56.***

"What will be the condition of the devotee who suffers from separation?" – asks Kabīr, and says that such a man does his duty (that can be performed with the body) vigorously and mediates on the bodiless Divine.

Note: The man who has not yet reached the "Kriyār para avasthā" goes on practicing Kriyā with vigor and tries to concentrate his mind on the Supreme Reality.

Kabīr yo jan birahī Nāmke, sadā magan man māñha
Yyo darpaṇ ki sundarī, kāhu na pakari bāñha. ***57.***

Kabīr says that the person suffering separation from the Holy Name is constantly engaged in recalling the Lord and sometimes goes to catch Him. His attempt, however, is as fruitless as that of a man trying to catch the reflection of a beautiful lady in a mirror.

Note: The devotee has a constant hankering after the Divine. The Divine is there in the body within the Kûṭastha, but so long as one does not reach the "Kriyār para avasthā" one cannot be united with Him.

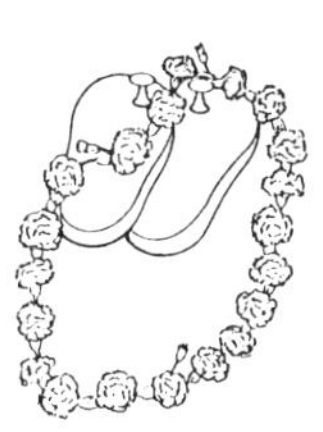

Chapter - 10

Wisdom and Separation

Kabīr cingi āgki, mo tan pari urāy
Tan jvarike dhartī jvari, āor jvare ban rāy. ***1.***

Kabīr says: "A spark of fire has burnt my body and even the best of forests has been burnt up."

Note: Constant practice of Prāṇāyāma – burns all the desires which are at the root of all grief.

Kabīr dīpak pāyoak āniyā, tel bhariā āsang
Tin milike joiyā, uṙi uṙi paṙe patang. ***2.***

Kabīr says that the lamp is burning with oil and fire. It is the combination of these three things, viz., the lamp, oil and the fire, which keeps the lamp burning. But because of earthly attachment, the mind, like an insect, is being burnt up.

Note: The lamp is a symbol of the Kûṭastha, the two-petalled lotus within the forehead. The fire is the Light Divine seen through Kriyās within the Kûṭastha. The oil stands for the Jīvātmā or the human consciousness. The devotee sees the Light Divine in the Kûṭastha as a result of his practice of Kriyās, and gradually his earthly attachment wears off in contact with the Holy Light just as an insect dies in contact with fire.

Kabīr hirdayā bhitar dvo bāre, dhuñyā nā pargaṭ hoy
Yāki lāi so lakhe, ki yihna lai Samyoy. ***3.***

Kabīr says that two lines of fire are burning in the Kûṭastha, although there is no smoke. But he is unable to see him for whom he had concentrated his gaze in the Kûṭastha.

Note: The two lines of fire denote the two ganglias – Īṛā and Pingalā. So long as the Prāṇa-Vāyu (vital breath) flows through these two channels, the mind remains restless with earthly attachment. Smoke is an indication of fire. But the speciality of the gangliated cords of sympathetic nerves is that their activities are without any prior indication. It is often seen that a man becomes conscious of a wrong-doing only after the deed is done. That is why the burning (activity) of the Īṛā and Pingalā has been described as without smoke. They are also unable to lead us to the Supreme Lord. It is only when (through Prāṇāyāma) the Prāṇa-Vāyu flows through the Suṣumnā, the subtle passage through the spinal cord, that our mind is enabled to concentrate on the Divine.

Kabīr mārā hāy so mari geyā, Brahma Agni ki bhāl
Mūrakh koi jāne nehi, catur lakṣe sab Kheyāl. ***4.***

Kabīr says that he who was attacked with the spear of Divine fire has been dead. Ignorant people do not understand this, but wise men see everything.

Note: If we attack the restlessness of our minds with a sincere practice of Kriyās, the restlessness will vanish after a time and a steady attention to the Divine will gradually take its place.

Kabīr mārā hai mari yāyegā, binā sāng ki bhāl
Parā pukārai birich tar, āju mare ki kālha. ***5.***

Kabīr says that he who was attacked with the bladeless spear has been crying from under the tree. He will die today or tomorrow.

Note: The mind has been made steady with Kriyās and so the restlessness has almost died out. But till the "Kriyār para avasthā" is reached, and the Divine reveals Himself in full splendor, a complete annihilation of the mind is not possible.

Kabīr coṭ santāoye biraha ki, Sab tan jhañjar hoy
Mārni hārā jānchi, ki yis lāgāye hoy. ***6.***

Kabīr says that the devotee, separated from the Divine, has been suffering intense pain and the entire body has been full of pores. The Jīvātmā, who is inflicting the pain, is conscious of it. But the Paramātmā seems to be totally unconcerned.

Note: So long as the Sādhaka does not transcend the bodily consciousness and become one with the Supreme Lord in the "Kriyār para avasthā", he has to suffer intense pain and anguish.

Kabīr jhal uṭhi sakalo jvarā, khapar phuṭā sañjut
Hamsā Yogī ramī geyā āsan rahi bibhūt. ***7.***

Kabīr says that the Divine Fire has burnt everything. Even the top portion of the head seems to have burst. The Yogī who was tasting the union with the Lord, has disappeared; only his seat and powers remain.

Note: The Yogī in the "Kriyās para avasthā" becomes completely detached from his body. His consciousness becomes one with the Supreme. But so long as he lives in this mortal world, his body still remains the seat of the Divine and a source of miraculous powers for doing good to humanity.

Kabīr āgi lāginī rame, kāñdo jvaria jhāri
Utar dakhiṇ kā paṇḍitā, mare vicāri vicāri. ***8.***

Kabīr says that water, by catching fire, has been burnt up; even the mud has been burnt. Scholars are only wasting their time in arguments on North and South.

Note: Water here denotes the Jīvātmā or the human conciousness, and mud stands for our sense-organs. The Divine fire of Kriyā leads them gradually away from the world of attachment. But as the devotee proceeds along the path of detachment, worldly-wise men condemn him by all sorts of useless arguments.

Kabīr dvau lāgi sāyer jvarā, macchi jvariā āy
Dādhe jīv na ubre, Satguru gaye lagāy. ***9.***

Kabīr says that the water-tank has been burning for the two (Īṛā and Pingalā), and the fish, too, has been burnt. Although the Sadguru has applied his instructions, the burnt man has not yet crossed over to the new world.

Note: Due to practice of Kriyās, the mind moves away from the Īṛā and Pingalā and enters into the Suṣumnā. The mind has been described as a fish. As the Prāṇa-Vāyu flows through the Suṣumnā as a result of Kriyās, the mind gradually becomes dead to the mundane consciousness. But so long as it is not completely merged in

Divine consciousness in the "Kriyār para avasthā", the devotee does not reach complete Self-Realization.

Kabīr Guru dagbhā celā jvalā, biraha jāgāyi āg
Tinukā bāpurā ubrā, Guru pūre ki lāg. ***10.***

Kabīr says that both Guru and disciple have been burnt and the fire of separation is burning still. The Sadguru has been the cause of all this fire.

Note: The ego of the devotee has been referred to here as the disciple, and the Jīvātmā or human consciousness as the Guru. But the Jīvātmā is often being united with the Paramātmā, and the individuality of the devotee has been surrendered before the Divine. Both have therefore been described as burnt down. But the devotee has not yet settled in the Supreme Consciousness, and therefore the yearning continues. The root cause of the entire process has been the Sadguru.

Kabīr āhari sanga lāgiyā, mrgā pukārai roy
Yehi ban hām krīṛā kiyā, dābat hāy ban soy. ***11.***

Kabīr says: "The deer as well as the hunter are both lamenting loudly that the forest in which they used to play is being burnt."

Note: The mind has been compared to a deer, and the human consciousness which generally controls the mind has been compared to a hunter. With advancement in the practice of Kriyās, the mind and the human consciousness itself gradually merge in the Divine Consciousness. This has been described as the death of the hunter as well as the deer. The endless desires of man have been described as a forest. But as the devotee advances towards "Kriyār para avasthā", desires are gradually annihilated.

Kabīr mai ghar jvārā āpnā, liyā lukāyā hāth
Ar ghar jvāro tāhikā yo lagai hamāre sāth. ***12.***

Kabīr says: "I have burnt down my own house with a torch in my hands; and whosoever will accompany me will have his house burnt by me."

Note: The torch here refers to the Kûṭastha or the Divine Effulgence. With the practice of Kriyās the devotee himself has reached the Kûṭastha, and he will now lead others to the same state of Divinity.

Kabīr paṭṭan śāṛī jvar geyā, dhāgā ek nā dādh
Ghar siñṛi, pagṛī kaṣā, parā kuṭum bādh. ***13.***

Kabīr says that the silk cloth with all its threads has been completely burnt up. Using the stairs within the body, he has reached the top and caused obstruction for his relatives by tying his turban tight.

Note: The thoughts of the brain have been spoken of as a silk cloth. In the "Kriyār para avasthā" all earthly thoughts are merged in Divine Consciousness, and hense the silk cloth has been described as burnt up. For reaching the "Kriyār para avasthā", the devotee has to cross the six plexuses, described as the six stairs in the body. But once he reaches the "Kriyār para avasthā" in the Sahasrāra, he never allows the physical organs to control him.

Kabīr ghar jvāre ghar ubre, ghar rākhe ghar yāy
Ek ācambā dekhiyā, muā kālko khāy. ***14.***

Kabīr says that when the house is burnt, it flourishes; but when it is carefully looked after, it falls down. He has seen a miracle, that a dead man has devoured up Time.

Note: When the Fire of Kriyā burns down earthly attachment, the devotee reaches the permanent shelter of Divine Consciousness in the "Kriyār para avasthā". But pre-occupation with earthly desires never leads one to perfect bliss. A man who has reached the Transcendent Consciousness is, to all intents and purposes, dead to the world of mundane reality. But it is he who has reached the Life Eternal. Since he has overcome restlessness through the Kriyās, he has reached a state of complete tranquillity and his consciousness is no more affected by the passage of Time. It is in this sense that he has triumphed over and devoured up Time.

Kabīr sorṭhā Samundar lāgi āgi, nadīyā jvāri kaylā bhayi
Dekha Kabīrā jāgi, macchi tarioyar coṛi geyi ***15.***

Kabīr says that the sea has caught fire and the river has been burnt up into coal. The fish has climbed up to the tree. Seeing all this, Kabīr has awakened.

Note: Our desires have been compared to Oceans and rivers. The body is the tree, and the "Bindu (Divine Consciousness) is the fish. With advancement in Kriyās, the desires are gradually burnt, i.e., annihilated. The Consciousness reaches the 'Sahasrāra', and then alone the devotee wakes up into a life Divine.

Kabīr āge āge dvau bāre, pache hariyarā hoy
Balihāri uyā brch ki, yā jari kāṭe phal hoy. ***16.***

Kabīr says that at first there is a separation between the Jīvātmā and the Paramātmā. Later they are turned into one. Thanks to that tree, which, even when cut at the root, never fails to yield the fruit.

Note: With long practice of Kriyās a time will come when the human consciousness will be merged in the central dark point of the Kûṭastha. The consciousness, when uprooted from earthly desires, will bear the fruit of Divine Bliss.

Kabīr biraha kul hāṛi tan bahai, ghāo na bādhai roha
Marṇe ki śamsai nahi, chuṭī gayā bharam moha. ***17.***

Kabīr says that the axe of separation has run over the body, and therefore there is no doubt about death. All errors and illusions have disappeared.

Note: Kriyā is the art of merging human consciousness with the Divine. Although it means much labor on the part of the devotee, the labor ultimately destroys all earthly illusion and attachment.

Kabīr swapanā raiṇakā, parā kare ye chek
Yab śoyo tab dui janā, yab jāge tab ek. ***18.***

Kabīr says that when he dreams within his sleep, he has a dual consciousness. But when he is awake, he is one.

Note: The earthly consciousness is like a dream beside the Supreme Reality. At this stage, due to lack of union between the human and the Divine Consciousness, the two remain two. But in the "Kriyār para avasthā", there is complete union between the Jīvātmā and the Paramātmā and hence the One alone exists.

Kabīr pāni māhi par jvali, bhayi aparbal āgi
Saritā bahati rahi geyi, mīn rahe jal tyāgi ***19.***

Kabīr says that the fish remains within water, but its fins are burnt. Fire has no force now. The river has stopped flowing. The fish has come out of the waters.

Note: The fish is the mind. The water is the Primal cause or Brahman. The two fins of the fish are the Īṛā and Pingalā, the two sympathetic nerves. During the practice of Kriyās, the mind, leaving the Īṛā and Pingalā, enters the Suṣumnā. Then, in the "Kriyār para avasthā", the mind loses itself in the Divine. There is no more any flow of the Prāṇa-Vāyu, no restlessness whatsoever.

Kabīr Brahma agni tan mo lāgi, lāgi rahā tata jīu
Ki jāne oha birahiṇī, ki jāne O Piu. ***20.***

Kabīr says that the Divine Fire has caught the body and the jīva (human consciousness) sticks to the Fire. This is being felt by the Jīvātmā whose Samādhi has been broken up by the beloved Lord.

Note: The human consciousness, in the "Kriyār para avasthā", can no more remain attached to the body; it gets lost into the Divine Fire. But the devotee, in the initial stages of the "Kriyār para avasthā", cannot always remain in that state of complete absorption. Whenever that state is broken, he feels intense pain.

Kabīr pāvak rupī Rām hāy, sab ghaṭ rahā samāy
Cit cakmak cin haṭāy nahi, dhūñā hoy hoy yāy. ***21.***

Kabīr says that the Lord is the Fire, and He stays in every body. The Consciousness sticks to that Fire and merges its existence there just like smoke gradually losing itself in the fire.

Note: The 'Citta' or subtle human consciousness – slowly merges itself into the Divine, with prolonged practice of Kriyās.

Kabīr kar kāyā cakmak kiyā jhārā bārambār
Tin bār dhūñā bhaya, cauthe parā angār. **22.**

Kabīr says that he has struck the flint of the body repeatedly. Thrice it was only smoke, and in the fourth time it became a piece of burning charcoal.

Note: When anybody concentrates his gaze in the Kûṭastha, in between the eye-brows, he at first sees nothing but darkness; then, gradually, the Kûṭastha reveals itself in various pleasing colors.

Kabīr pahileñ Prem na cākhiā, mujhe niraśī āy
Pācheñ tan man hāt lay, gaye camkā lāy. **23.**

Kabīr says that he was at first disappointed without any taste of Love. Later on, however, as the mind and body were controlled, he had the taste of the wonderful.

Note: Due to delay in Self-Realization, the devotee practicing Kriyās gets disappointed. Later on, however, he experiences the desired thing.

Kabīr birahā mujh soñ eoñ kahe, gārā pākṛo mohi
Caraṇ kamal ke mojme, lai bayṭhāoñ tohi. **24.**

Kabīr says that Separation has told him also this: "Catch me tight, and I shall make you sit at the Lotus-Feet of the Lord."

Note: If Somebody practices Kriyā, he will gradually reach the "Kriyār para avasthā."

Kabīr āguyāni to āiyā; jñān bicār bibek
Pāche Haribhi āiya, sagari sāj sāj samet. **25.**

Kabīr says that the predecessors, – Wisdom, Analysis and Conscience – have come first. Later comes the Lord Himself with all his paraphernalia.

Note: As a result of practicing Kriyās, the devotee experiences the presence of the Lord within the Kûṭastha.

Chapter 11

On Familiarity (With the Divine)

Kabīr tej Anantkā, yyāysā Sūruj sayan
Pati sang jāgi Sundarī, Kautuk dekhat nayan. ***1.***

Kabīr says that the glow of the Brahman is like that of the Sun which has just set – neither light nor darkness. The feelings aroused by the manifestation of the Brahman (the Divine) within the body are like those of a beautiful lady keeping awake for union with her husband and feasting her eyes with his sight.

Note: The Divine Effulgence manifested within the Kûṭastha is indescribable. It ravishes the body and mind of the devotee in the "Kriyār para avasthā".

Kabīr Parabrahmake tejkā, kyāysā hāy anumān
Kyā oyāki śobhā kahoñ, dekhan ki parmāṇ. ***2.***

"How can the Divine Splendor be guessed?" – asks Kabīr . "How can its beauty be described? One has no means of realizing this, unless one has direct experience."

Note: The Divine is really indescribable. He can only be felt in the "Kriyār para avasthā".

Kabīr agam agocar gami nahi, tāñhā jhalke jyoti
Tāñhā Kabīrā bandogi, pāp puṇya nahi dvauti. ***3.***

Kabīr says that he has bowed down to the Supreme who is unapproachable by sense-organs as well as by human intelligence. He is shining in His own Light and in Him there is no dichotomy of sins and purity.

Note: The "Kriyār para avasthā" is the Transcendent state of Consciousness which is above ordinary comprehension. It is a state where there is not yet any separation between joys and sorrows, purity and impurity. It is an absolute state of monism, where duality simply does not exist. This state of Consciousness, however, can only be reached through a prolonged practice of Kriyās.

Kabīr man madhukar bhayā kiyā nirantar bās
Kñaol yo phulā nirbic, ai nirakhe nija Dās. ***4.***

Kabīr says that the mind has been like a bee and resides constantly in the Lotus (within the head), which is the Source of all knowledge. This, however, is experienced only by a servant of the Ātmā or the Divine.

Note: Through the practice of Kriyās, the mind ultimately is merged in the Sahasrāra (the thousand-petalled lotus within the head), the special seat of the Divine within the human body.

Kabīr chip nehi, Sāgar nahi, Svātī bundbhi nāhi
Kabīr moti nipje, śūnya śikhar gaṃmāhi. ***5.***

Kabīr says that there is no oyster, no ocean, no drop of water when there is the star Svātī in the sky; and yet the pearl is shining in vacuum.

Note: It is said that if a drop of rain is devoured by an oyster when the star Svātī rises in the sky, a pearl is formed within the body of the oyster. In the present context, the pearl is the white dot within the Kûṭastha which can only be seen through the practice of Kriyās.

Kabīr ghāṭme āoghāṭ pāiyā, āoghāṭāyoñ hi ghāṭ
Kahe Kabīr parce bhayā, Guru dekhāi bāṭ. ***6.***

Kabīr says that he has now discovered an āghāṭā (a place where there are no paved stairs for reaching a tank or river for purposes of taking bath) within the ghaṭ (a staircase leading to a tank or river). He has recognized the āghāṭā as the proper ghaṭ. It is the Guru who has shown him this proper path.

Note: The normal breathing has been described as a paved stairway and the "Kriyār para avasthā" as an āghāṭā. We shall have to reach the "Kriyār para avasthā" for achieving liberation from bondage. For this, however, the guidance of the Sadguru is essential.

Kabīr yāñhā matihuki jhālrī, hīrhuko pargāś
Cāñd Sūrya ki gami nahi, tāñhāñ darśan pāoye Dās. **7.**

Kabīr says that not even the Sun and the Moon can enter the place which is studded with pearls and glowing like diamonds. But the servant of the Divine has a passport to that region.

Note: The Divine Light which presents itself before the devotee with the practice of the "Yonimudrā", has innumerable pearl-like drops and the splendor of diamonds. It is the Light Divine which is the prime source of all light – even that of the Sun and the Moon. But the man who surrenders himself before the Sadguru has an easy access to that Light which is brighter than innumerable Suns and yet cooler than the rays of innumerable Moons. Surrender and not egotism is the way to success in Kriyās leading to Divine Consciousness.

Kabīr Sūrya Samānā Cāñd me, dvau kiyā ghar ek
Manko cītayo gayā, pūrba janamkā lekh. **8.**

Kabīr says that the Sun and the Moon have united to make one single room. The restlessness of the mind is no more; and the fruits of works of the previous births have been annihilated.

Note: In the advanced stage of Kriyās the Īṛā (the Sun) and the Pingalā (the Moon) – the Sympathetic Nerves – are united at the root of the Suṣumnā within the forehead. The mind of the devotee becomes tranquil; and due to union with the Divine, the devotee has no more to suffer the pangs of earthly attachment.

Kabīr piñjar Prem pragāśia, antar rāhā ujās
Mukh Kasturī maha mahiñ, bāṇī phuṭi subās. **9.**

Kabīr says that the cage of Love has been revealed, but it can only be felt within. This is just like musk kept within the mouth. The fragrance of the musk cannot be smelt by others excepting when the man with the musk speaks.

Note: If a man practices Kriyā with love, his Consciousness becomes encaged as it were; because it can never again stay away from the Divine.

Kabīr Yogī huye yak lagi, meṭi gei at cātān
Ulṭi Samānā āpume, hoy gayā Brahma Samān. ***10.***

Kabīr says that he has become a Yogī. But he remains like a miser. All his desires have been annihilated. And he has come to be like Brahman, although he remains within himself in the opposite posture.

Note: The greatest wealth of the human being is the latent Divine Energy in the Mūlādhāra. The Yogī, by means of Kriyās, makes this Energy unite with the Divine in the Sahasrāra. This is the opposite process of the normal earthly activities. Once, however, the Yogī is Conscious of this greatest treasure within himself, he no more allows his mind to stray away from this. Thus, jealously guarding the Supreme possession, the Yogī can be compared to a miser in a sense.

Kabīr kachu karaṇī kachu karma gati, kachu pṇrbilā lekh
Dekho bhāg Kabīr kā, kiā dost ālekh. ***11.***

Kabīr says that due to some good work (Kriyā) in this life and also in the previous births, he has now been fortunate enough to acquire friendship with the Invisible (the Divine).

Note: Practice of Kriyās through many births ultimately leads man to "Kriyār para avasthā" when he is united with the Divine.

Kabīr kāyā chip Samsārme, pāni buñd śarīr
Binā chip ki moti, pragaṭe dās Kabīr. ***12.***

Kabīr says that this world is like an oyster and the body is like a drop of water. But the pearly dot in the Kûṭastha comes without any connection with the oyster.

Note: Kriyā leads the human mind gradually away from earthly Consciousness. The white dot within the Circle of Light seen through the Kriyās, therefore, does not depend on the outside world.

Kabīr yoha moti yani jānahu, yo poye poni sāth
Eha to moti śabdaki, yo bedhi rāhā sabh gāt. ***13.***

Kabīr says: "Dọn't put your mind to earthly attachment; put it rather to the Divine Sound 'Ohm' which vibrates throughout the body. Devour up evil propensities just as you do it in case of a piece of bread."

Note: Due to practice of Kriyās the sound 'Ohm' becomes audible to the devotee. His mind is gradually concentrated in that sound.

Kabīr man lāgā unmunī soñ, gagan pahucā yāy
Cāñd bihunā cāñdnā tāñhā alakh Niranjan Rāy. ***14.***

Kabīr says that when the mind is merged in the vacuum (in the Sahasrāra), it reaches the Brahman. The place of the Brahman is there where there is moonlight but no moon.

Note: In the "Kriyār para avasthā" there is no separate existence of the mind. It is merged in the supreme in the Sahasrāra.

Kabīr man lāgā unmunī soñ, unmum manahi bilag
Loṇ bilagā paniyā, pāni loṇ milag. ***15.***

Kabīr says that whenever the mind reaches the Brahman, it becomes separated (from earthly attachment). The salt was separate from the water, but now it has melted into the latter.

Note: The Brahman is like a vast ocean and the mind is like salt. In the "Kriyār para avasthā" the human mind no more remains attached to earthly things but gets merged in the Divine.

Kabīr pānihuñte puni hem bhayā, hemo geyā bilāy
Kabīrā yo thā soi bhayā, āb kachu kahā nā yāy. ***16.***

Kabīr says that the water became gold, but the gold again has vanished. The original situation has come back and nothing need be said.

Note: The mind has been compared to gold which is a precious thing. Originally, there was no separate existence of the human mind or Consciousness, because there was nothing else but the Lord. But as soon as individual Consciousness developed, through the Will of the Divine, the mind got engaged not with the

Divine but with His Creation consisting of varied and beautiful things. Just because man gets much earthly satisfaction with the mind, it has been described as gold. But through a long practice of Kriyās the mind again gets merged with the Divine in the "Kriyār para avasthā." In this state of Self-Realization man gets back to his original home, viz., the Divine.

Kabīr Surati kañol me baiṭhke, amī saroyar cākh
Kañhe Kabīr bicār kai, tab Śanta bibekī bhākh. ***17.***

Kabīr says: "Take your seat on the lotus of good desires and taste the juice from the tank of nectar". The considered opinion of Kabīr is that such tasting, however, can only be done by men of conscience who have already achieved tranquillity.

Note: It is only he who has reached the "Kriyār para avasthā" who can taste permanent bliss.

Kabīr adhar kañolke upre, parimal śvet subās
Amī kañoyal par baiṭhike, darśan daraś hu lās. ***18.***

Kabīr says that he enjoys great Bliss by seeing mystic visions, sitting on the lotus of nectar situated above the lips and within the white and fragrant piece of cloth.

Note: The blooming of the lotus of nectar happens when the devotee experiences innumerable visions in the Kûṭastha.

Kabīr abigat ki gati kyā kahoñ, yāke gāño na ṭhāño
Guṇ bihunā dekhiye, kyā kahi dhariye nāo. ***19.***

Kabīr says: "What shall I say of the motion of him who is immovable? By what name should I call Him who has neither any residence nor any characteristics?"

Note: God is realized in the "Kriyār para avasthā" which is a state above all motion and characteristics.

Kabīr oyāki gati ās alakh hāy, alakh lakhā nehi yāy
Śabd Svarūpī Rām hāy, sab ghāṭ rahā samāy. ***20.***

Kabīr says that since the Supreme is beyond our physical vision, His movements are also invisible. The Sound "Ohm" is Rāma (the Lord), and He is present in everybody as Sound.

Note: The most complete realization of the Divine can only be had in the "Kriyār para avasthā". But since the mind itself is non-existent in that state of Consciousness, who will see the movements of the Supreme Reality?

Kabīr yeñhi kāraṇ hām yātthe, soi pāyā ṭhāor
So to pheri āpnā bhayā, yāko kahate āor. ***21.***

Kabīr says that he has now got the address of Him for who he started his voyage. Kabīr used to consider himself separate from the Lord, but now the Lord has become his own.

Note: In the "Kriyār para avasthā" there remains no distinction between the human consciousness and the Divine, for the two get completely identified.

Kabīr māy jāno yo milonge, koi āor Rāmko dhāy
Āpu ramiyā hoi rāhā, śīṣ noyāo kāy. ***22.***

Kabīr says: "If I could know beforehand that I would have to be united with my own Self. I would not run after the Lord (Rāma) as distinct from myself. When I have been identified with Rāma before whom should I bend my head in obeisance?"

Note: In the "Kriyār para avasthā" the devotee gets identified with the Divine.

Kabīr maṭuk manohar adhik chabi, bhed nā pāoye koy
Banknolko sam karai, Gugugam kahiye soy. ***23.***

Kabīr says that the picture is more beautiful than the Crown, but the distinction is known only by him who can unite his tongue with the Kûṭastha through the Grace of Shriguru.

Note: The mind has been described as the crown. But the Kûṭastha, which has been described as a picture, is more attractive than the mind. In order to reach the Kûṭastha the devotee has to take his tongue to a particular position which can only be taught by a great master of Kriyāyoga.

Kabīr yāñhāñ paon nāhi sañcāre, tāñhā raci ek graha
Acaray ek yo dekhiyā, siñddha kalejā deha. ***24.***

Kabīr says: "I have built a house where there is no motion of the air. But I am surprised to find a great change of my heart and the whole body."

Note: "Samādhi" (a state of complete absorption in the Divine) is an absolutely tranquil state of consciousness when the heart and even the entire body become still and motionless.

Kabīr ḍhāṛhas dekho cakor ki, siñddha kalej dinha
Hirdayā bhitar paiṭhike, lāl ratan Hari linha. ***25.***

Kabīr says: "See the guts of the curlews. They have pierced the heart and got the precious jewel there."

Note: The two eyes are like two birds, fixing their gaze on the third eye, i.e., the Kûṭastha. Through the Kriyās the attention of the devotee gradually goes inwards and is fixed on the Divine. The 'heart' in Yoga often means the two-petalled lotus (in between the eye-brows), the gateway to the kingdom of heaven within our body.

Kabīr alakh lakhe lālac lago, kahat bane nahi bayan
Nija man dhaso svarūpmo, Satguru dinhe Śayan. ***26.***

Kabīr says: "When the Unseen becomes visible, the devotee becomes full of hankering. But he can no more relate his experience, because he gets completely absorbed in the Supreme Self through the Grace of the Sadguru."

Note: It is through the Grace and guidance of a great spiritual Master that we can have Self-Realization (i.e., God-Realization). But once we have it, we have no power to express the experience in words.

Kabīr unman lāgi sunyamo, niśu din rahe gul tñān
Tan man ki kachu sudhi nahiñ pāyā pad nirvāṇ. ***27.***

Kabīr says that on reaching the highest experience, he felt a sort of a vacuum. His throat was choked and he had no sense of the body or mind. It was thus that he reached "Nirvāṇa".

Note: On reaching the "Kriyār para avasthā" we are completely free from bondage, the bondage of all earthly desires. "Nirvāṇa" literally means elimination. It is in the highest stage of spiritual experience that we are free from even our bodily limitations and become living souls.

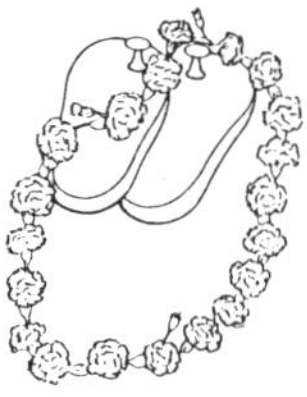

Chapter 12

On Restlessness

Kabīr pyāylā Premkā, antar liyā lagāy
Rom Rom me rami raho, amal na āor so hāy. ***1.***

Kabīr says that the cup of Love has touched the heart and has given each pore a ravishing joy. As the love increases, the joy, too, knows no end.

Note: In the "Kriyār para avasthā," the Prāṇa-Vāyu becomes still in each pore of the skin and this is a state of perfect Divine Love and Divine Bliss. Anybody who practices to remain in this supreme state of Consciousness, has a longer and longer duration of such moments, and consequently, greater Bliss.

Kabīr Hari ras eo piyā, bāki rahim chāk
Pākā kalas koñ bhārkā, bahuri caṛe nahi cāk. ***2.***

Kabīr says that one who has drunk the juice of Hari (the Lord), has no hankering after taking anything else; just as a burnt jar has no more any necessity of being put on the fire by the potter.

Note: A man who, by prolonged practice of Kriyās, has reached perfect union with the Divine in the "Kriyār para avasthā" and is a permanent settler in that state of consciousness, gets completely liberated from the bondage of repeated births and deaths.

Kabīr Rām rasāyan adhik ras, piyoto adhik rasāl
Kabīr pion so durlabh hāy, māge śīṣ kalāl. ***3.***

Kabīr says that Rāma (the Lord) is the greatest medicinal drink and one who takes to Him, becomes full of nectar. But it is very difficult to have a sip of that nectar, for, in order to do it, one must cut off one's head.

Note: To cut off one's head here means to lose one's ego completely. In order to be thoroughly absorbed in Divine Bliss in the "Kriyār para avastā", one must completely surrender one's ego before the Lord. For this, the discipline of the Kriyās is an absolute necessity.

Kabīr bhāñṭi Prem ki, bahutak baiṭhe āy
Śir sope pioye soy, āor so piyā na yāy. ***4.***

Kabīr says that the Elixir of Love Divine can only come after long practices. And he alone who can offer his head is able to drink this Elixir.

Note: "Bhāñṭi" means the pan in which something is boiled. Beneath the pan there is fire. Here the pan is the human body in which the fire of Kriyā generates the Elixir of Divine Love. Only when, due to long practices of Kriyā, the Prāṇa-Vāyu gets settled within the head (in the Sahasrāra), the devotee experiences complete Bliss. This is what has been described as offering the head itself to the Divine.

Kabīr Hariras mahaghāñ jānikai, māge śīṣ kalār
Dil oñccā ghanṭ dublā, baiṭhike gāoye mālār. ***5.***

Kabīr says: "The Elixir of Hari (the Divine) is very dear. One has to offer one's head first in order to taste it. But the body is weak, and the heart is bad. Now, therefore, there is no other way but to sing in the Mallāra tune."

Note: The word "Hari (the Lord) literally means "One who takes away" (our ego). In order to reach Hari or the Supreme state of Consciousness one has to go beyond the physical Consciousness. But the body is weak, it is not always fit for hard practices of Kriyās through which alone the Supreme Reality can be reached. The heart, too, is often unable to take resolve for a determined progress towards the Divine. "Mallāra" is a tune which, sung aright, would call forth rains which cool down earth. In order to cool down his restless nerves the devotee bides time till his body and mind become fit for hard practices in Kriyās. This biding time has been described as singing the Mallāra tune.

Kabīr Hariras māhange piyatā, choṅ jīvanki bāṇ
Māthā sāṭe Ṣāñi mile, tao lāgi sulabh jān. ***6.***

Kabīr says: "If you want to taste the Elixir of Hari (the Divine Bliss), abandon all hopes of your life: Only when you chop your head off, the Lord will be easily available to you".

Note: To offer one's head means to remain in the "Kriyār para avasthā" all the time. It is only then that the nectar of Divine Bliss can be had.

Kabīr abadhūtā ābi gatirahitā, yyāysā akhil ajit.
Nām amal mātā rahe, jīvanmukti atīt. ***7.***

Kabīr says that the "avadhūta" (the Saint) has overcome all restlessness. He has dropped all desires for conquering anything in this Universe. He is drunk with the "Amal" (the Lord, in whom there is not an iota of dross), and has become free even in this human life.

Note: The man who is constantly in the "Kriyār para avasthā" is free from all bondage, from all desires, and has completely transcended the mundane Consciousness.

Kabīr āṭ gāñṭ kopīnme, manahi nā āne śank
Nām amal mātā rahe, kāñhā Rājā kāñhā rank. ***8.***

Kabīr says that there are as many as eight knots in the loin-cloth of the Saint. He has no fear in his mind. He is constantly absorbed in the Name of the "Amal". Who is the king for him and who the "Fakir" (a mendicant)?

Note: The Saint has no shame even if his slender garment is torn into pieces and knotted together in many places. He is not afraid of anything. He is constantly in the "Kriyār para avasthā". Since he has no desire to have anything, he makes no difference between the king and the Sannyāsin. He wants neither riches from the king nor spiritual power from a sage. He is absorbed in the Bliss of Self-Realization.

Kabīr Hariras piyā tar jāniye, utre nehi khoyāri
Mātoyālā ghumat phire, tan ki nāhi samāri. ***9.***

Kabīr says that a man who is drunk in "Harirasa" (the Divine Elixir, the Divine Consciousness) has no respite from his

Intoxication. He roams about like a mad man, without any body-Consciousness.

Note: The attainment of the "Kriyār para avasthā" makes one indifferent to all earthly considerations, including physical ones.

Kabīr yoñha sar ghaṙā na ḍubtā, maygal mali mali nāhāy
Deol ḍubā kalas so, parkhat Sāñi yāy. ***10.***

Kabīr says that even a pitcher cannot be drowned in the water of the tank. And yet a man takes his bath in it and washes the dirt from his body. The temple (i.e., the human body), as well as the pitcher (i.e., the head) gets drowned. But once you want to see, it is no more.

Note: The limited human Consciousness has been likened to a tank with meager water. At this stage the devotee experiences difficulty even in practicing Prāṇāyāma. But once he reaches the transcendent stage, he is one with the Ocean of "Saccidānanda" in which the whole body and mind, and everything else is immersed. In this "Kriyār para avasthā" he has no separate human identity to see whether all movements of his mind have actually stopped. If he wants to investigate it, he has to disassociate himself from the Divine and come downwards from the "Kriyār para avasthā".

Kabīr sabhe rasāyan māy Kiyā, Hariras āor na koy
Rancak ghaṭme sañcare, sab tan kāncan hoy. ***11.***

Kabīr says: "I have tasted all kinds of juices; but it is only when even the smallest quantity of the Divine Elixir enters the body that the entire constitution is transformed into gold. This transmutation cannot be made by any other thing."

Note: In the "Kriyar para avastha" the entire body gets charged with the Divine.

Kabīr ekantha chāk chakāiya, ekantha piyā dhoy
Kal kalanti bhāṭhi yinha piyā rāhā kāl leñ śoy. ***12.***

Kabīr says that the devotee who drinks the Divine nectar for the second time, after properly filtering it, is lying with Time (or Death).

Note: When the "Kriyār para avasthā" comes to the devotee for the first time, it does not always last long. But again, when through practices of the Kriyā, the Sādhaka reaches it, he becomes Timeless, one in his Consciousness with the Eternity.

Kabīr kahat śunat jag yāt hāy, bikhayan śujhe kāl
Kaheñ Kabīr re Prāṇiyañ! Bāṇī Brahma Sañbhāl. ***13.***

Kabīr says that the world is moving fast while we go on seeing and listening. The gall of earthly possessions does not allow us to see Time. "O creatures!", Says Kabīr, "Hold the word of Brahman (the Lord), i.e., the Sound Ohm".

Note: Doing this and that is merely wasting time. The only worthwhile activity is to go on controlling the breath i.e., practicing Prāṇāyāma which would ultimately lead us to the sound of "Ohm". Listening to this sound, one gradually settles down in the "Kriyār para avasthā".

Kabīr rato mātā Nām kā, piyā prem aghāy
Mātoyāle didārke, māge Mukti balāy. ***14.***

Kabīr says that the Sādhaka (devotee) becomes intoxicated with the Name of God. He drinks Love to the throat and neglects even liberation from the body.

Note: The "Kriyār para avasthā" is a God-intoxicated state when even 'Siddhi' (success in spiritual practices) seems to be insignificant.

Kabīr rato mātā Nāmka, madkā mātā nāhiñ
Madkā mātā yo phire, se mātoyārā nahi. ***15.***

Kabīr says that the Saint has been drunk with God's Name. But this drunkenness is not like the intoxication produced by alcoholic drinks which makes one talk nonsense. The Divine intoxication keeps one absorbed in his own Self.

Note: The "Kriyār para avasthā" is a state of Divine drunkenness. The sage remains completely absorbed in Self-Realization at this state and feels no attachment to anything in this world.

Kabīr mātoyālā ghumat phire, rom rom bharipūr
Choṭe āś śarīr ki, tab dekhe dās Hajur. ***16.***

Kabīr says that the God-intoxicated man roams about, with every pore of his skin full of that intoxication. It is only when the servant (the devotee) is completely devoid of attachment to his body, that he is granted a vision of the Master (i.e., God).

Note: The "Kriyār para avasthā" generates a complete indifference to physical considerations.

Kabīr Prem piyālā bhari piyo, jar nā karo yatan
Āyo chāk yab jānsi, sohāge dharo ratan. ***17.***

Kabīr says: "Take cupfuls of Divine Love. Do not have any slackness in taking it. Since you have recognized it after filtration, stick to the Kûṭastha which is like a jewel".

Note: Filtering Divine Love means removing all material grossness that might remain mixed up with our hankering after the Divine. We can experience Love in its purity only when our mind gets fixed in the Kûṭastha.

Kabīr bhauñrā bāri parihari, maṙi bilanme āy
Pāvan candan ghar kiyo, bhuli gayā bānarāy. ***18.***

Kabīr says that the black bee, leaving water, has taken shelter in a hole. Taking shelter within sandalwood, it has forgotten the King of the forest himself.

Note: Although the proper resting place for man is the Divine, he generally remains forgetful of his Maker. Practices of Kriyās lead him again to the Divine.

Kabīr amṛt keri, rākhi Satguru choṙi
Āpu Sarikhā yo mile. tāhi piyāoye ghori. ***19.***

Kabīr says that the Sadguru has kept the nectar separate and when he comes across a kindred spirit, he shakes it well and makes the latter drink it.

Note: The Sadguru makes the sincere devotee taste the nectar of Divine Bliss in the "Kriyār para avasthā".

Kabīr amṛt piye so janā, yāke Satguru lāge kāṇ
Oyeto agocar mil goy, man nahi āoye ān. ***20.***

Kabīr says that he who is all ears to the Sadguru drinks the nectar. He has realized the unknown and his mind does not deviate to anything else.

Note: The Sadguru makes the sincere disciple listen always to the sound of "Ohm" which leads him to the "Kriyār para avasthā". Once he reaches that stage, he has no more any attachment to anything but the 'Brahman' (the Supreme).

Kabīr Sādhu chip hāy, Satguru Svāttī bund
Tṛkhā gei ek bundte, Kyā le kare Samund. 21.

Kabīr says that the sincere disciple is like an oyster and the Sadguru is like the raindrop fallen from the sky when the star Svātī is there. Since all thirst is quenched by that single drop,what use the Ocean would now be?

Note: The pearl grows within the oyster only when it absorbs a drop of rain when the star Svātī is ascendant in the sky. So also Divinity gradually reveals itself to the disciple when a man with Self-Realization (the Sadguru) initiates him with the spiritual process (Kriyā). The drop of rain is symbolic of the "Kûṭastha", the fixed point where the disciple has to concentrate his mind. The Ocean full of waves symbolizes the restlessness of all earthly things as contrasted with the steadiness of the Divine.

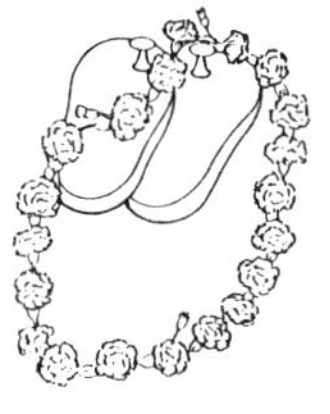

Chapter - 13

On Steadiness

Kabīr kāyā kaonḍal bhari liyā, ujal nirmal nīr
Piyat trkhā na bhājal, tirikhāvant Kabīr. ***1.***

Kabīr says that he has filled in the jug of his body with bright and pure water, and yet his thirst is not quenched.

Note: The Brahman is Illimitable, and therefore, even when one is full of the Divine Bliss, one hankers after more of it.

Kabīr man ulṭā dariā milā, lāgā mali mali snān
Thāhat thāha na pāiya, tirikhā rahi amān. ***2.***

Kabīr says that the mind has got into a river where the current comes from the opposite direction. There it takes a dip and washes itself thoroughly. Kabīr has not been able to fathom the depths of the water, and yet his thirst remains equally strong.

Note: The opposite current is the movement of the Kula-Kuṇḍalinī (the Latent Divine Energy in every human body) upwards towards the head, as a result of the devotee's practice of the Kriyās. The devotee takes his bath as it were in the river of Kriyās, and, gradually, his mind gets more and more purified, till he reaches the "Kriyār para avasthā" which is Illimitable and unfathomable Bliss.

Kabīr panḍit se ti kahi rāhā, kāhā na māne koy
Āo gāhā eha ko kahe, bhāri ācaray hoy. ***3.***

Kabīr says that he has narrated his experience to worldly-wise persons, but they do not believe his words. When he invites them to the same experience, they only wonder.

Note: Without initiation from a Sadguru, it is not possible for a man to have an experience of the Divine.

Kabīr jore base eha tan maha, tā gati lakhe na koy
Kahe Kabīrā Santa jan, baṛā acambhā hoy. ***4.***

Kabīr says that nobody (in the ordinary world) is able to see the Presence (of the Lord) who takes a forcible occupation of the body and resides there. Only Saints see Him in amazement.

Note: The presence of the Divine within the body can only be seen through the Kriyās.

Kabīr ghaṭme rahe śujhe nahi, karaṇ soñ śunā na yāy
Milā rahe āo na mile, tā soñ kahe basāy. **5.**

Kabīr says that the Lord is within the body, and yet nobody understands Him, nobody hears Him, nobody gets united with Him. How, therefore, would one make one's consciousness steady in him?

Note: The Divine cannot be experienced with the help of physical organs. It is only through the Kriyās that our Consciousness can reach Him.

Kabīr karaṇ kahe karṇe śune, bhanak pare nahi kāṇ
Yyāse sant na ha sutise, pāohi Brahma ginān. **6.**

Kabīr says that one says and hears through the ears, but ordinary sounds are of no use. The Saints realize the Brahman through the sound of "Ohmkāra".

Note: The dumb are generally deaf. One does not say anything unless one can hear. The worldly people therefore listen through their ears and speak. But the ears can give them only the earthly sounds. The unearthly sound "Ohm" comes through the Kriyās and it is through this inner sound that the mind of the devotee gets gradually absorbed in the Divine.

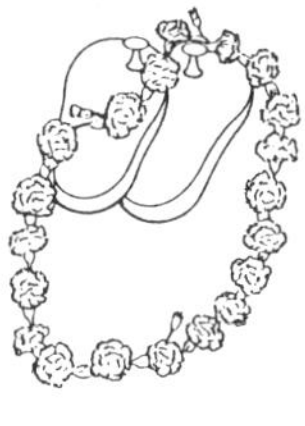

Chapter - 14

The Vision

Kabīr herata herata he sakhi, herata gai heray
Bund samānā sindhume, so kita herā yāy. ***1.***

Kabīr says: "O friend! while searching for you, search itself is lost. The speck is lost in the Ocean, how can it be found any longer?"

Note: The individual human consciousness is completely merged in Divine Consciousness in the "Kriyār para avasthā".

Kabīr herata he sakhi, rāhā Kabīrā herāy
Sindh samānā bundme, so kita herā yāy. ***2.***

Kabīr says: "O friend! while searching for you, Kabīr himself is lost. Since the speck is lost in the Ocean, how should anyone search for that?"

Note: The speck of light at the Kûṭastha (the point in between the eye-brows) is replaced, through the Kriyās, by the resplendent all-pervasive light of the Divine.

Kabīr bund Samānā Sindhume, so jāne sabh loy
Sindhu samānā bundme, bujhe biralā koy. ***3.***

Kabīr says that everybody knows that the speck enters the ocean, but very few know that the Ocean too enters the speck.

Note: The "Kûṭastha bindu" (the speck or dot of light seen within the Ājñā Cakra) is actually the miniature Brahman. But this can be realized only in the "Kriyār para avasthā" when the devotee has experienced the vast Ocean of Divine Consciousness.

Kabīr samudra samānā bundme, gau khurke asthān
Iccārūp samāiya, bahuri na pāoye jān. ***4.***

Kabīr says that as the Ocean has entered the speck, the latter looks like the hoof of a cow. The mind enters within that space and then becomes totally indifferent to all earthly affairs.

Note: When, by fixing one's gaze in between the eyes, one reaches the "Kriyār para avasthā", one's Consciousness always remains above the mundane plane of reality.

Kabīr ek samānā sakal me, sakal samānā tāhi
Kabīr samānā bujhime, yāñhā dosro nāhi. **5.**

Kabīr says that the One has entered everything and everything has entered the One. Kabīr himself entered the One, where there is no second.

Note: The Brahman or Paramātmā is all-pervasive. That everything and everybody is Brahman (The Lord in His impersonal aspect) is realized in the "Kriyār para avasthā" when the devotee knows that the Supreme Reality is One and without any second.

Kabīr Guru nahi celā nahi, nahi murid nahi Pīr
Ek nahi duja nahi, tāñhā bilme dās Kabīr. **6.**

Kabīr says that he takes rest in a place where there is no Guru nor disciple, no Pīr (Muslim Saint) nor his disciple, where there is not even one – not to speak of two.

Note: "Kriyār para avasthā" is indescribable, because there is no distinction between the knower and the knowable in that state of Consciousness. The devotee himself, i.e., his human Consciousness, is totally lost in the Divine. This is a state of perfect tranquillity and ultimate rest for the human mind.

Kabīr birchayo ḍhuñṛe bījkoñ, bīj birchake pāhiñ
Niojo ḍhuñṛe Brahmako, Brahmajioke māhi. **7.**

Kabīr says that the tree searches for the seed, but the seed is there within the tree itself. So also everybody seeks the Brahman, although Brahman is there within everybody.

Note: The source of all creation is Brahman. He is the seed, and the Universe comes from Him. But He cannot be realized without Kriyā or spiritual practices.

Kabīr ādī hatā so ab hāy, pher phar kachu nāhi
Yeño tariorke bījme, ḍār pāt phal chāñhi. **8.**

Kabīr says that what was there in the beginning continues to exist even now. It does not know any change; just as the seed contains within itself the leaves and branches, the fruits as well as the shade given by the tree.

Note: The Supreme Reality is unchangeable. It remains the same in past, present and future. Since it is the source which contains germs for everything, the devotee has to realize this Source through Kriyās.

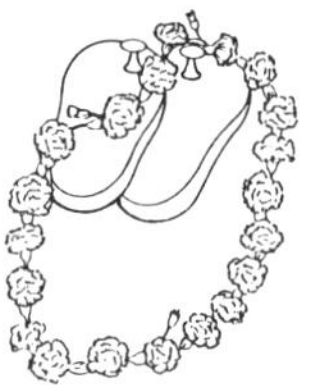

Chapter - 15

On Attaining Immortality

Bhārī Koho to bahu ḍareñ, hālukā kaho to jhuṭ
Me nehi jāno Rāmko, diṣṭa dekhā nahi muṭ. ***1.***

Kabīr says: "If you call Him (the Lord) heavy, I become afraid. If you call Him light, that will be falsehood. I do not know Rāma (the Lord), for if I could keep Him within my grip, then alone could I see Him."

Note: The Lord is heavier than the heaviest and lighter than the lightest. His nature cannot be described in words. That is why, even when Saints realize Him, they cannot set any limits to that Illimitable Reality.

Kabīr diṭhā hāy to kyā kaho, kahoñ ta ko pati āy
Hari jyāche tyāche rāhā, tum harkhi harkhi guṇ gāy. ***2.***

Kabīr says: "If I say that I have seen Him, who will believe me? I am also unable to describe Him in words. Hari (the Lord) remains as he is. Let us only sing His praise."

Note: The Brahman cannot be expressed in words, even when one realizes Him in the "Kriyār para avasthā".

Kabīr yyāchi kathani mati katho, kathone dharo chapāy
Ved kiteboñ nā likho, kahoṇ ta ko patiyāy? ***3.***

Kabīr says: "Do not talk about the Supreme Reality. Rather maintain secrecy about Him. Do not try to establish Him in books, for who will believe your words?"

Note: Mere words are useless in attaining Realization. Practicing Kriyās is the surest way to reach the Supreme Reality.

Kabīr kartā ki gati āor hāy, tu cal apne anumān
Dhīre dhīre pāo dharu, pañhuce gā nija ṭhām. ***4.***

Kabīr says: "The movements of the Lord are independent of your speculations. What you should do is to be guided by your own capabilities. You should move on with wary steps and reach your own place."

Note: After a prolonged practice of Kriyās, the devotee reaches the "Kriyār para avasthā," when he will be united with the Lord; and that is man's proper resting place and real home. Before that he can only go on practicing Kriyās to the best of his capacity.

Kabīr pañhucoge taba kahahuge, ab kachu kāhān yāy
Ajahu bhelā samudrame, boli bigāṛe kāy. **5.**

Kabīr says: "When you actually reach there, you will say that you have nothing to say and really nothing can be said. The boat is still in mid-Ocean. Let it reach the opposite shore first and then have words. Otherwise your words may not be correct."

Note: Before reaching "Kriyār para avasthā" anything that we say about the Divine may be incorrect. After reaching that stage, however, the Saints feel that they cannot express the indescribable Reality.

Kabīr jāni bujhi jaṛa hoy rahe, bal teji nirbal hoy
Kaheñ Kabīr tehā Dāsko, pāllā na pakṛe koy. **6.**

Kabīr says that one who has understood (the Supreme Reality), becomes still. In full possession of (Divine) strength and vigor, he does not make a show of them. Kabīr says that ordinary people cannot gauge the depths of such a man.

Note: When Kriyā purifies the mind, one becomes Self-absorbed and cannot indulge in idle talks.

Kabīr bād bibād bīkhay ghanā, bole bahut upādhi
Mauna rūp gahi Hari bhaje, yo koi jāne sādhi. **7.**

Kabīr says that unnecessary talks only increase material attachment and titles. He who has really known Hari (the Lord), worships Him silently.

Note: To go on practicing Kriyās without indulging in idle talks is the path of progress towards the Divine.

Kabīr Sākṣi ek Kabīr ki, śuni śikhi nahi yāy
Rañcak ghaṭme sañcare, tau ajar amar hoy jāy. 8.

Kabīr says that it is not necessarry to have faith in his evidence. Once you experiment and establish the Divine within yourself, you will be immortal.

Note: Mere faith in the evidence of sages will not do. What is essential for Self-Realization is to practice Kriyā.

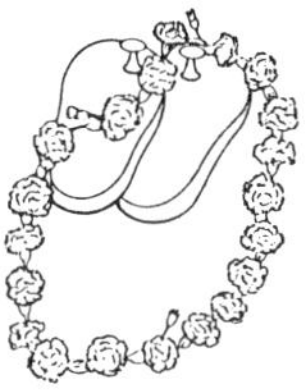

Chapter - 16

The Location (of the Divine within the body)

Kabīr surati tekuri lau lejurl, man niti dār nihār
Kaula ku āmi Prema Rasa, pīoye bāram bār. ***1.***

Kabīr says: "Take out the thread from the spindle with calmness of mind and fix your mind in that. You will then be able to drink the nectar of love that is there within the lotus?."

Note: The spindle stands here for the Kûṭastha and threads are the spiritual experiences. When one fixes one's mind in the Kûṭastha, one will drink the juice from the Sahasrāra, the thousand-petalled lotus within the head.

Kabīr Gangā yamunā ke antare, sahaja śūnya hāy ghāṭ
Tāñhāñ Kabīrā maṭ racoñ, Muni jana jo-oye bāṭ. **2.**

Kabīr says that there is a vacant field in between the rivers Gangā and Yamunā. Kabīr has built a temple over there, and the sages want to go to that place.

Note: The Sympathetic Nerves – Īṛā and Pingalā are often descirbed in the Scriptures as the Gangā and the Yamunā. The Suṣumnā (the subtle passage within the spinal cord) is generally described as the river Sarasvatī. Sarasvatī is the goddess of learning. The Suṣumnā, through practices of Kriyāyoga, leads the devotee to Self-Realization. The Suṣumnā ends in the Sahasrāra where there is a vacuum (measuring ten fingers placed side by side). It is this seemingly vacant place which is considered to be the highest seat of God within the human body. The human consciousness, when it reaches this place, gets completely merged in the Divine.

Kabīr jehi banśi ghana Sañcarai, Rāi panchi nā uṛi āy
Moṭā bhāg Kabīr kā, tāñhā rāhā lau lāy. **3.**

Kabīr says that when the sound of the reed grows intense, Rādhā, like a bird grows, spell-bound and does not fly away. Kabīr has concentrated his mind intensely in that sound.

Note: Śrī Rādhā was the greatest devotee of the Lord when He manifested Himself as Lord Kṛṣṇa on earth. The term Rādhā here has been used symbolically in order to mean the devotee. She has also been compared to ạ bird spell-bound by the sound of the flute made by Lord Kṛṣṇa. The musical sound referred to here is the 'Anāhata Nāda', the subtle sound which can be heard after long practices of Prāṇāyāma. Absorption in the Nāda gradually leads one to Self-Realization.

Kabīr lao lāgi tab jāniye, kabhi choṙi na yāy
Jīyat to lāgi rahe, muye māhi samāy. ***4.***

Kabīr says that once there is identification with the Divine, it is never lost. It lasts as long as the body, and after destruction of the body in death the devotee gets completely merged in Brahman.

Note: Once the devotee attains perfect control of the 'Kriyār para avasthā', it is never lost. Even after death it leads him to complete merger with the Divine.

Kabīr yyāchi lagi yo raso, tyāychi nim hāy choṛ
Koṭi Koṭi jorike, Kiyā lākh karor. ***5.***

Kabīr says that as the devotee gradually tastes the Divine nectar, attachment to worldly objects seems to him as bitter as margosa. Tasting thus the Divine juice crores (ten millions) of times, he attains permanent Bliss.

Note: With repeated practice of Kriyāyoga, the 'Kriyār para avasthā' becomes permanent.

Kabīr yyāychi upje peṛ soñ, tyāychi nim hāy jor
Āpne tan ki kyā kahai tāre paribār karor. ***6.***

Kabīr says that as the margosa tree (bitter nim, i.e., lack of worldly attachment) grows stronger and stronger, the devotee grows more and more indifferent to his own bodily comforts and becomes the means for liberating innumerable souls.

Note: As the 'Kriyār para avasthā' settles permanently, the devotee becomes a sage, a Sadguru who is able to train men and women in the processes of Kriyāyoga, the way to commune with the Divine.

Kabīr yyāychi prathame lau lagai, tyāychi dhurle yāy
Yāke hirday lau basai, so mohi māhi samāy. ***7.***

Kabīr says that the hankering after union (with the Divine) should be kept up till the last stage when the devotee has complete Self-Realization.

Note: The eagerness for practicing Kriyās should be continued till we settle in the 'Kriyār para avasthā.'

Kabīr jar lagi kathani ham katho, curi rāhā Jagadīś
Lau lāgi pai nā pare, ab bola nā nahi Dīśa. ***8.***

Kabīr says: "So long as 'I' (i.e., my human self) go on talking the Lord remains at a distance. But at the time of merging of my limited self with Him I do not have any desire to speak."

Note: The separate consciouness of the human self is annihilated in the "Kriyār para avasthā".

Kabīr satguru taṭu lakhāiā, grantha hi māhi mūl
Lau lāgi niramal bhayā, meti gayā samśay śūl. ***9.***

Kabīr says that the Sadguru has shown the process. But the Supreme Source is within the body itself, and the consciousness, due to its union with the Divine, has become purified, and the doubts have all been dispelled.

Note: As we proceed along the path indicated by the Sadguru by means of practicing Kriyās, our consciousness in the "Kriyār para avasthā" gets purified and free from doubts.

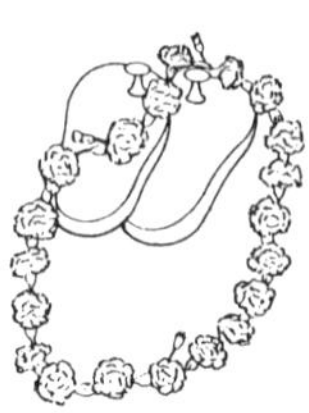

Chapter 17

On Chastity

Kabīr prit lāgi meri tujhte, bahu guṇia lay kanta
Yao hāñsi boli āor te, to nitahi rangāyo danta. ***1.***

Kabīr says: "I have developed great attachment to you, for you are a lover with innumerable qualities. When I used to laugh and talk with others, I would color my teeth in order to look beautiful.

Note: Due to constant practice of Kriyās Love Divine grows within the heart of the devotee. At this stage his behavior with everybody becomes sweet and tender.

Kabīr caitti rahoñ na bisaroñ, tu pada daraśi thāy
Eha anga bañdaro bhalā, yab tujh soñ miliyā āy. ***2.***

Kabīr says: "Please keep me always in your mind, and make me always keep my mind at your Lotus Feet. Even if my body becomes like that of a monkey, let me remain united with you. Otherwise everything is useless for me."

Note: Our attention should always be there in the Kûṭastha till we can merge completely in the "Kriyār para avasthā".

Kabīr nayhā bhitar āu tuñ, teñha nayan jhapehu
Nahi dekha āor koñ, nā tu dekha na dehu. ***3.***

Kabīr says: "Please come within my eyes. My eyes are shut when you come. At that time my eyes are unable to see anybody else. You, too, do not allow me to see anybody."

Note: Due to prolonged practice of Kriyās, the gaze of the devotee becomes constantly fixed on the Divine till at last in the "Kriyār para avasthā" everything seems to be a manifestation of the Divine.

Kabīr rekhā ek sindūr ki, kajrā diyā na yāy
Nayanan Rām rācār hāy, dujā kāñhā samāy. ***4.***

Kabīr says: "There is a mark of vermilion in the eyes, so collyrium cannot be given. 'Rāma' has already been there in my eyes, how should a second come in?"

Note: The flame of light of the Kûṭastha has been compared to a line made by vermilion, and worldly objects have been compared to collyrium when the devotee has constant union with the Divine, he cannot have any earthly attachment.

Kabīr āt pahar causaṭ ghare, mere āorān koi
Nayananha me tum hi baso, nid na āoye soi. **5.**

Kabīr says: "I am all alone throughout the twenty-four hours. There is nobody else with me. As you have placed yourself on my eyes, I have no wink of sleep."

Note: When at the primary stage the devotee gets concentrated in the Kûṭastha, his mind sometimes is diverted to other things. But gradually his concentration becomes permanent. As there is no break in his union with the Divine, his consciousness does not have any rest or sleep.

Kabīr nid dekha yab purṣako, ulaṭi āpu uṭhi yāt
Tāte nikat āoye nehi, mūrhan te na derāt. **6.**

Kabīr says: "When the human consciousness sleeps, (in the 'Kriyār para avasthā'), it turns upside down automatically, and does not come back to its former position. At this stage there is no fear which has normally to be faced at the stage of imperfect consciousness."

Note: In the "Kriyās para avasthā" there is no separate human consciousness. Everything becomes Brahman at this stage. Hence, there is no fear or anxiety.

Kabīr sāñi mere ek tu dujā āor na koy
Dujā sāñi tab kaho, yab kali Dujā hoy. **7.**

Kabīr says: "You alone are my Lord, and there is no second for me. One may talk of a second lord only when there are two separate buds."

Note: Before union with the Divine, there seem to be two separate selves: the Jīvātmā and the Paramātmā. In the "Kriyār para avasthā" however, the Jīvātmā gets merged in the Paramātmā and there is One Single Existence.

Kabīr bārbār keyā, āñkhiyā, mere man ki śoy
Kalito uthali hoygi, sāñi āor na koy. ***8.***

Kabīr says: "What else should I see repeatedly with my eyes? The Lord lies in my own mind. When the bud will bloom, I must see Him, for there is none else but He for me."

Note: The Divine is the only Master for man. One should seek union with Him through the Kriyās.

Kabīr balihāri oyā duhkha ki, yo pal pal Rām kāhāy
Oyā sukhkhe māthe śila, yo Hari hirdayā so yāy. ***9.***

Kabīr says: "Glory be to such grief which makes us take the Name of Rāma every moment. Shame to such happiness which makes us forget the Name of Hari."

Note: The strain for practicing Kriyās is a blessed one, for it leads us ultimately to the union with the Divine in the "Kriyār para avasthā."

Kabīr rahe samudrako bīcmo, raṭe piyās piyās
Sakala samudra tinukā gaṇe, ek Svātī bund ki āś. ***10.***

Kabīr says: "While floating on the Ocean, I have yet to cry out in thirst. Just because I am waiting for the 'Svātī drop of water' (the drop of rain while the star Svātī is ascendant in the sky), I consider the sea-water as no better than grass."

Note: Worldly life has been compared to an Ocean and the Paramātmā to the Svātī drop. The man practicing Kriyās can never be completely satisfied till he reaches identification with the Divine in the "Kriyār para avasthā."

Kabīr sukh kāraṇ ko yāt the, āge miliyā dukh
Yāhu sukh ghar āpne, hāmre duhkha samukh. ***11.***

Kabīr says: "I was seeking for happiness but it is grief which has come first. The home for happiness is within myself, but grief lies in my front."

Note: One has to pass through the strain of practicing Kriyās first before one can hope to attain the "Kriyār para avasthā."

Kabīr dojak to hām angayā, so ḍarā nāhi mujh
Bihinti na merto cāhiye, bāñjhu plyāre tujh. ***12.***

Kabīr says: "Although Hell covers all my limbs, I have no fears. I do not want (worldly) happiness or grief. I want you, O my beloved! Even if I have to go fruitless (childless), I want none but you."

Note: 'Bāñjha' or 'Bāñjhu' means one with no son or daughter. It is part of worldly happiness to have children. But although children are dear to us, the dearest is the Lord Himself. All around us is the dirt of worldly life, but if we go on practicing Kriyās, we shall not be affected by that filth, and in the "Kriyār para avasthā' we shall be united with our beloved Lord.

Kabīr yo ohi ek na jāniā, to sab hi jān ajān
Yo ohi ek hi jāniā, to sabe ajān sujān. ***13.***

Kabīr says: "He who does not know the One, even if he knows many things, knows nothing. He who knows the One, even if he knows nothing, knows everything."

Note: One who has knowledge of the Self through Kriyās, becomes Omniscient, for there is nothing in this Universe or beyond this but the Self or the Supreme. Without Self-Realization there may be knowledge in different subjects like Literature, Physics, Chemistry, etc., but such knowledge can only be partial and fragmentary and cannot lead one to liberation.

Kabīr yo oha ek na jānia, tao sab jāne kyā hoy
Ek hiñte sab hoñt hāy, sab te ek na hoy. ***14.***

Kabīr says: "What avail all kinds of knowledge if the One is not known? It is because the One remains, the many exist. But the many cannot produce the 'One'."

Note: It is because God is everything, to realize Him (God-Realization is just another name for Self-Realization) in the "Kriyār para avasthā" would enable us to see "into the life of things".

Kabīr ek sādhe sab sādhiā, sab sādhe sab yāy
ulṭike siñce mul koñ, tao phule phale aghāy. ***15.***

Kabīr says: "Service to One would mean service to all. But service to everybody would mean service to nobody. When the root, placed upside down, is watered, the tree becomes full of blossoms and fruits."

Note: To concentrate the mind on the Divine through Kriyās is the best spiritual exercise. A mind diverted towards different purposes is the source of all troubles. The root of the body is within the head. As contrasted with the root of a tree, it stands in the opposite direction. It is not the lowest part of the body, but the highest. That is why Kabīr says that the root, turned upside down, should be watered. Watering the root would mean to satisfy God by means of Kriyās (devotional practices).

Kabīr sab āyā us ek ko, ḍār pāt phal phul
Kabīr pācheñ kyā rāhā, yab pakrā nija mūl. ***16.***

Kabīr says: "Everything has sprung up from the One: leaves and branches, fruits and flowers. When I have clutched the root, what remains to be caught?"

Note: Once there is union with the source of the Universe in the 'Kriyār para avasthā', everything is achieved.

Kabīr mūl Kabīrā gahi caṛe, phal khāyā bhari peṭ
cor sāhuki gami nahiñ, yeño bhāoye teo leṭ. ***17.***

Kabīr says: "Clutching the root I climbed up the tree and ate fruits to my heart's content. Thieves and men addicted to riches cannot reach there. Whatever occurs in the mind of the person who reaches there, comes true."

Note: Men with worldly addictions cannot reap the fruits of Supreme Consciousness. But anybody who reaches that

Consciousness in the "Kriyār para avasthā" has complete fulfillment in his life.

Kabīr yao man lāgay ek soñ, tao niruāri yāy
Sādar doy mukh bājati, ghana tamā bākhāy. ***18.***

Kabīr says that when the mind gets concentrated, the channel opens up. But when one indulges in mere talks, one has to pass through many difficulties.

Note: God-Realization cannot be attained through mere idle talks. One has to concentrate one's mind in the Divine through Kriyās.

Kabīr āśā to ek nām ki, cuji āś nirāś
Pāni māhi ghar kiyā, soko mare piyās. ***19.***

Kabīr says: "The only expectation that can be made is that of the Divine's Name. The second hope is of attaining a hopelessness (i.e., desirelessness). I have built my house in water, and yet I have to go without water."

Note: At first we should want the 'Kriyār para avasthā.' At this state, everything becomes a manifestation of the Divine and therefore no earthly desire remains.

Kabīr kali yug āike, kiyā bahut so mit
Yinha dil bāṇdhā ek soñ, tinha sukh pārā nit. ***20.***

Kabīr says that the Kali Yuga has come and tried repeatedly to make friends (with the devotee), but it could not do any mischief to the man whose mind has been bound to the One. Such a man is in possession of eternal happiness.

Note: Kali Yuga or Dark Age symbolizes sins and vice. Yuga means 'double'. When the breath flows through Īṛā and Pingalā, the two gangliated cords of sympathetic nerves the mind remains restless and prone to vices. But he who has concentrated his gaze in the Kûṭastha, has his breath flowing through Suṣumnā, the one single passage leading to the Supreme One. He will never again be disturbed by evil.

Kabīr patirbartā ko sukh sanā, yāke barat hāy ek
Man mayli bibhcāriṇī, tāke khasam anek. ***21.***

Kabīr says: "A chaste lady has great happiness, for she has single-minded devotion. But she whose mind is dirty is unchaste. She has many masters."

Note: One whose mind is in the Kûṭastha has the Divine as her only Master. But anybody who does not concentrate in the Divine suffers from varied and conflicting desires.

Kabīr patibartāko ek hāy, bibhcāriṇī ko doy
Patibarat bibhcāriṇī, kahu ko bhala hoy. ***22.***

Kabīr says that the chaste is one, but the unchaste are two. Who is better between the chaste and the unchaste?

Note: The Suṣumnā (the subtle passage within the spinal cord through which the breath must pass in order to lead a spiritual life) is one, but the Īṛā and the Pingalā are two. It is always better to canalize the vital breath through the Suṣumnā with the help of Prāṇāyāma.

Kabīr patibartā mayli bhali, kāli kucili kurūp
Oyāke mayle rūp par, oyāro koṭ svarūp. ***23.***

A chaste lady, even if she is black and ugly, is better than crores of handsome but unchaste women.

Note: Concentration in the Divine is better than all kinds of talents.

Kabīr patibartā tab jāniye, rati na khaṇde nayan
Antar soñ sāñc rahe, bole miṭhi bayan. ***24.***

Kabīr says: "A woman may be called truly chaste when her mind never deviates from the husband even for a single moment. She is sincere at heart and sweet in her words."

Note: A real devotee remains always concentrated in the Divine. Since he knows everything and everybody as manifestations of the Divine, his behavior cannot be rough and rude.

Kabīr bāle bhole khasam ki, bahut kiyā bibhcār
Satguru rahe batāiyā, Param Purukh bhartār. ***25.***

Kabīr says: "In my young age I indulged in many acts of unfaithfulness due to ignorance. But after having guidance from the Sadguru I have known the Lord of the Universe to be my husband."

Note: Before having Self-Realization through Kriyās man does not have continuous absorption in the Divine. But when the 'Kriyār para avasthā' settles permanently on him, his consciousness never deviates from the Lord.

Kabīr bhed yo leoye baithī kyo, sab soñ kahe pukāri
Dharā dhare so dharkuṭī, adhare dhare so nārī. ***26.***

Kabīr says: "He who has understood the essence proclaims loudly before all that one having easy access from the Mūlādhāra (the lowest plexus) to the Sahasrāra achieves a permanent position of rest. But one who catches only the lips remains a woman."

Note: With continued practice of Kriyās one has an easy access to the Divine within the head through the Suṣumnā. This can never be achieved with the help of intoxicating drugs taken through the lips.

Kabīr myay sevak sāmarath ko, koi pūrabkā bhāg
Śoyat jāgi sundari, Sāñi diyā sohāg. ***27.***

Kabīr says that he is a worshipper of the state of Equality. This has been due to his good fortune of the previous births. The beautiful lady who was so long sleeping has now awakened and the Lord has given her His favor.

Note: Due to practice of Kriyās in many births it becomes possible for the devotee to attain the state of neutrality (above and beyond all restlessness) or the "Kriyār para avasthā." To attain this the kula-kuṇḍalinī or the Latent Divine Energy in the human body (compared to a sleeping lady) is to be awakened and united (through Kriyās) with the Divine (the Lord-lover of the lady) within the head.

Kabīr myay sevak sāmārath kā, kab hi naho akāj
Patibartā nangī rahe, tao ohi piyākoñ lāj. **28.**

Kabīr says that he is a worshipper of the state of Neutrality and therefore he never does anything wrong. Even if a chaste lady remains naked before her beloved, she does not feel ashamed. It is rather the husband who feels the shame.

Note: Nothing wrong can ever be done by a man who remains in the "Kriyār para avasthā." Such a man becomes a Saint. But if a devotee's mind does not always rest in the Brahman, he will commit some wrongs for which the Lord Himself will feel ashamed.

Kabīr tu tu kahe to dūri ho, dūri kahe to āo
Yyo hi rākhe tyo raho, yyo deoyā so khāo. **29.**

Kabīr says: "If you consider Him to be very near to you, He may be far away. On the other hand, if you think of Him as far off, He may be very near. Stay as He keeps you, eat what He grants."

Note: The man who reaches "Kriyār para avasthā" surrenders himself completely to the will of the Almighty.

Kabīr yo gāoye so gāoyia, yo joṛe so joṛ
Patibartā āo sādhu jan, eha Kali mahañ hāy thor. **30.**

Kabīr says: "Anybody who sings may be called a singer (whether he is good at singing or not). So do your work as you can. In the Kali Yuga (Dark Age) chaste ladies and Saintly persons are rare."

Note: Since goodness is very rare in the modern world, even a man who has just been practicing Kriyās according to his capabilities (and has not yet attained 'Siddhi' or consummation) may be appreciated as a Yogī, just as anybody who sings may be called a singer.

Kabīr Paramesur āye pāhuna, śunya sane hi dās
Khaṭras bhojan bhakti karu, yo kabhi na choṛe pāś. **31.**

Kabīr says: "The Lord has come. His servant Kabīr has been with that Infinite. Make him taste all the six kinds of food (sweet, sour, bitter, pungent, saltish and astringent) and offer Him great devotion so that He never leaves your side."

Note: In all possible ways the devotee should surrender his own ego before the Divine, i.e., he should try to attain "the Kriyār para avasthā" where the limited human self is simply annihilated.

Kabīr uci yāti papihaya, naoye na nīcā nīr
Ki Surapati ko yācai, ki dukha pahe śarīr. ***32.***

Kabīr says: "The lark looks towards the sky and prays for showers from the clouds to the king of gods. Although there is ample water below (i.e., in the rivers and tanks), he does not drink it even when his life is at stake (due to intense thirst)."

Note: The devotee wants to taste the nectar oozing out from the Sahasrāra. But for that he has to take the strain of continued practice of Kriyās.

Kabīr myay abalā piu piu karoñ, nirguṇ merā piu
Śurya sanehi Rām binu, āor na dekho piu. ***33.***

Kabīr says: "I am a weak woman constantly calling my husband. My husband is infinite and above all qualities. Who can be His companion except 'Ātmārāma', i.e., one whose only joy is in union with the Supreme Self?"

Note: The devotee should surrender himself completely before the Divine, as a loving and faithful wife surrenders herself before her husband. Kriyāyoga leads him gradually to this complete surrender in the "Kriyār para avasthā."

Kabīr patibartā brata Kumbhajal, pati bhaji dhare biśvās
Andiśā citoye nahi, sadā yo piuki ās. ***34.***

Kabīr says: "The devotion of the faithful wife is as constant and without restlessness as a pitcher full of water. Her mind is fixed in her dear husband and never deviates to any other direction."

Note: The constant concentration of the devotee is in the Kûṭastha.

Kabīr patibartā, Kyāy rahe, yyāyse coli pān
Tab sukha dekhai piokā, yab cit nahi āoye ān. **35.**

Kabīr says that a faithful wife sticks to her husband as a brassiere sticks to the breast or the betel sticks to the mouth. Just because her mind does not move elsewhere, she tastes the happiness of union with her husband.

Note: Constant practice of Kriyāyoga makes the mind stick to the Divine.

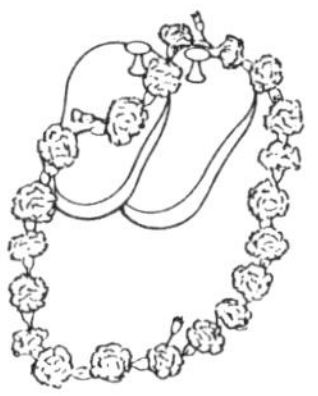

Chapter 18

For Realization

Kabīr naubat āpani, din daś lehu bājāy
Eha pūrā pāṭ na eha gali, bahurī na dekhahū āy. ***1.***

Kabīr says: "Let the bugle that is blowing within you blow for some (ten) days. Once you cross this stage, you do not have to come to it again."

Note: At a certain stage of the Kriyās the "Anāhata Nāda" or the sound of "Ohm" in its different varieties is heard from within the body. But this, too, is not the final stage of spiritual attainment.

Kabīr yehi ghar naobat bājti, myay gal bāñdhe doyār
Ekai Hari ke nām binu, gaye bajāoni hār. ***2.***

Kabīr says: "When the bugle blows, I attune my throat and doors (the inner ears) to its sound. But, ultimately, there is no other way but the Name of Hari (the Lord)."

Note: The mystic notes within are not sufficient for Self-Realization. The Name of the Lord here means the highest stage of spiritual consciousness which is indescribable, but which keeps the devotee in a constant rapture of union with the Divine.

Kabīr yinha ghar naobat bājti, hot chatiśo rāg
Te mandil khāli paṛe, baiṭh na lāge kāg. ***3.***

Kabīr says: "The room in which the music goes on with thirty-six different tunes will be vacant and crows will sit upon it."

Note: The stage in which the "Anāhata Nāda" can be heard is still lower than the "Kriyār para avasthā." If one cannot reach the "Kriyār para avasthā" one will not be liberated from the cycle of births and deaths. The room here indicates the body and it is only when the body is overtaken by death that crows sit upon it.

Kabīr ḍhol dāmāmā dundubhi sahanāi āru bherī
Ao sar cale bajāike, hāy koi lyāoye pheri. ***4.***

Kabīr says that a man might die while listening to the different Anāhata sounds like the sounds of double drums, kettle-drums large and small, tabors and flutes. But there are persons who, even after surpassing this stage, can bring it back in this very life.

Note: He who has reached the "Kriyār para avasthā" is a person who may be said to have died in the worldly sense. Although such a person has gone beyond the stage of listening to the Divine concert within, he can hear the sound whenever he wishes.

Kabīr thoṛā jīonā, māṛe bāhut manḍāṇ
Sab hi ubhā mel si, keyā rank keyā sultān. **5.**

Kabīr says that life is very short, but wanderings are many for everybody – the Prince as well as the pauper.

Note: Death will overtake everybody. So it is essential that we should not waste any time in useless activities. We should take to Kriyās seriously.

Kabīr ek din yyāysā hoyegā, sabhte pare bicho
Rājā Rāṇā chatrapati, sābdhān ko nahi so. **6.**

Kabīr says that a day will come when there will be separation from everybody. But the man who is in communion with the Divine will not have to suffer such separation.

Note: Death brings separation from everybody. But the man who is in "Kriyār para avasthā" comes to have an eternal consciousness which engulfs everything within itself. Since his consciousness becomes all-pervasive, whether in life or in physical death he is with everybody and at all time.

Kabīr ujar kheṛā thīkri, gaṛi gaṛi gaye kuñbhār
Rāoyaṇ sarikhā cali gayā, lañkāke Sardār. **7.**

Kabīr says that the Potter has made innumerable pots (here, human bodies) of brilliant colors. But although mighty figures like Rāvana the king of Lankā have disappeared, the Potter (the Supreme Self) remains the same.

Note: The creations change, but not the Creator. He, therefore, who has become one with the Unchangeable Creator in the "Kriyār para avasthā", has attained immortality of Consciousness.

Kabīr uñca mahal banāiya, cūṇe kali ḍherāye
Eke Harike Nām binu, yab tab pare bhulāye. ***8.***

Kabīr says: "I have built a high palace and white-washed it. But excepting the Name of the Lord I forget everything else."

Note: The high palace is the head where our consciousness reaches the "Kriyār para avasthā." At this stage nothing else interests us excepting the Name of the Lord.

Kabīr kañha garbiyo, lapeṭā hāṛ
Hayor upar chatrapati, tebhi dekhā khāṛ. ***9.***

Kabīr says: "How could you be proud with a body which is nothing but skin and bones? Only the king remains high up, overseeing everything?"

Note: The body is nothing but flesh and blood. Its only importance is that the Divine resides within it as the Omniscient Reality. Nobody, therefore, should be proud of handsome physical features, for they are transitory and will ultimately be transformed into the dust.

Kabīr kāñhāñ garbiyo, ucā dekhi āoyās
Kalhi paṛei bhuñi loṭnā, upar jāme ghās. ***10.***

Kabīr says: "Where should be your pride which makes you look so high? You will have to topple down the very next day on earth upon which the grasses will grow."

Note: Kriyā makes us realize the futility of all earthly pride.

Kabīr kāñhāñ garbiyo, kāl gañhe śir keś
Nā jāni kāñhāñ māri hāy, ki ghar ki pardeś. ***11.***

Kabīr says: "How could you be proud when time takes you by the forelock? There is no certainty as to where it will kill you – at home or abroad."

Note: Any moment we may die. Therefore it is essential to have our consciousness fixed in the Divine in the "Kriyār para avasthā."

Kabīr uttim kṣeti dekhike, garbe kāñhāñ kiṣāṇ
Ajahu jholā bahut hāy, ghar āoye tab jān. ***12.***

Kabīr says: "Does the peasant take pride on seeing a fertile land? You may see very good crops on the land to-day, but there may yet be many impediments on the way of harvesting them. It is only when the crops are safely brought home that the peasant is satisfied."

Note: We should not take pride after practicing a little of the Kriyās. It is only when we reach perfect tranquillity in the "Kriyār para avasthā" that we reach the desired goal.

Kabīr yehi ghar prīti na prem ras, āo rasana nahiñ Nām
Te nar āye samśar me, upaje kṣape bekām. ***13.***

Kabīr says: "A man having a house lacking in satisfaction and love and a tongue lacking God's Name is one who comes and goes in this world without any fruitful work."

Note: The house here is the human body. A man, after practicing Kriyās, should reach the "Kriyār para avasthā" and then he will be full of love for the Divine.

Kabīr yyāsā eha Samsār hāy, yyāysā mālatī phul
Din daśke beohār me, jhuñṭe rangan bhul. ***14.***

Kabīr says: "This world is like the Malati flower which for some time enchants man with its beauty and fragrance and then is no more. It deceives us with illusions for a short while."

Note: Since the earthly life is transitory, we should try to make its best possible utilization by practicing Kriyās.

Kabīr dhuri sakelike, poṭ bāndhi eha deha
Divas cārikā peknā, ant kheha ki kheha. ***15.***

Kabīr says: "This body is just like a bag of dust sent for a few days on this earth and then it merges into the dust again."

Note: The human body is evanescent.

Kabīr cāri pahar dhande gayā, tini pahaṛ rahu śoy
Ek pahar bandegi karo, yo janma saoyārath hoy. ***16.***

Kabīr says: "Four 'prahars (1 prahar = 3 hours) have been spent in so many works, and three prahars have been exhausted in sleep. But do not idly waste the remaining one prahar. Worship God during this period, and your life will reach its fulfillment."

Note: Even if one-eighth of the day and night is spent in practicing Kriyās, man may have Self-Realization.

Kabīr rāti goñyai śoi kari, divas goñyāi khāi
Hirā janma amol hāy, kauṅi bedleñ yāy. ***17.***

Kabīr says: "I have spent the night sleeping and the day eating. Life which is as precious as a diamond is being exchanged for a farthing."

Note: The precious human life should not be wasted merely in eating, sleeping and earning money.

Kabīr mandil khākkā jaṅā hī a lāl
Divas cārīk pekhnā, binaśi yāygā kāl. ***18.***

Kabīr says: "A day will come when his bodily temple will be burnt to ashes. It is in vain, therefore, that you are parading your diamonds and rubies. You have been sent here for a just few days, and then you will be destroyed by Time."

Note: However much we might value and decorate our body, it will ultimately be burnt to ashes after death.

Kabīr svapnāraiyankā, ughari gayā yab nayan
Jīu paṛā bahu luṭme, na cachu len na den. ***19.***

Kabīr says: "When the eyes open after dreaming, man becomes troubled with cares, for no give and take has been done."

Note: A time comes when man becomes worried that he has neither received Kriyā nor given it to anybody.

Kabīr i hāy citāoni, yau niruārī yāy
yo pahile sukh bhogīye, so pāche dukh khāy. ***20.***

Kabīr says: "A man who goes on enjoying earthly pleasures without the consciousness (referred to in the former verse), comes to grief in the ultimate analysis."

Note: A life without any attempt at Self-Realization, is destined to come to misery.

Kabīr āju ki kāl nahame, jangal hoyega bās
Upar upra ki rahenge, ṭhor caraṇ tā ghās. ***21.***

Kabīr says: "Your habitation will turn into a jungle sooner or later and you will have to roam about aimlessly on the grass."

Note: Sooner or later our bodies will be no more. So it is essential that we should practice Kriyās without wasting our time in idle pursuits.

Kabīr muye ho mari yāhuge, kai na legā nāo
Ujar yāi basāi ho, choṙi santā gāño. ***22.***

Kabīr says: "If you are dead, you will die. Nobody will remember your name. Leaving the residence of Saints, you will have to go somewhere else after your death."

Note: The man with earthly attachment is dead even in life. He will very soon be forgotten by the world, and, after his death, he will have to be born again with another body. But the man who remains in the "Kriyār para avasthā", absorbed in Divine consciousness, will be conquering death even when he shakes off his mortal frame." "He that believeth in Me (the Lord), though he is dead, yet shall he live. And whosoever liveth and believeth in me, shall never die."

Kabīr hāṛ jvare yeño lakṙi, keṣ jvare yeño ghās
Sab jab jvartā dekhi ke bhayā Kabīr udās. ***23.***

Kabīr says that the bones are burning like logs of wood, and the hairs are burning like grass. Seeing the world burning, Kabīr has become indifferent.

Note: Meditation on the transitoriness of everything in this world makes the devotee take shelter in the Divine Consciousness in the "Kriyār para avasthā."

Kabīr rākh nihārā bāhara, ciṙīyanha khāyā kṣet
Ādhā pardhā ubre ceti śake to cet. ***24.***

Kabīr says that when a man's attention remains diverted to the outside world, the birds eat up the harvest of his field. In order to prevent this, he should rise at least more than half his way (along the Suṣumnā) and then try to unite himself with the Divine.

Note: The body is the field where the harvest of Love Divine will have to be produced. But excessive material attachment of the mind is like birds who destroy the crops. This attachment is to be eliminated by prolonged practices of Kriyāyoga. When the devotee's mind rises at least up to the Ājñā Cakra, his earthly attachment is minimized to a great extent. If he continues his efforts even after that, he gradually reaches the "Kriyār para avasthā" in the Sahasrāra when he becomes completely one with the Divine.

Kabīr yo janme so bhi mare, hambhi cal nehār
Mere piche yo paṙā, tīnha bhi bāñdhā bhār. ***25.***

Kabīr says: "He who is born will die. I shall go away. But he who will come after me will also find an anchorage."

Note: Everybody who has not reached the Divine will have to die. Kabīr, since he has attained Self-Realization, will not have to be born again. Anybody who will go on practicing Kriyās will find a secure shelter in the Divine Consciousness.

Kabīr māy buṙhāni bāp buṙhānā, ham bhi mājh buṙhāy
Keotiyāke nāo, yeño, samyoge mile āy. ***26.***

Kabīr says: "My mother has been drowned, my father also has followed suit. I myself was drowned in their midst. But fortunately a fisherman's boat has rescued me."

Note: Prakrti, i.e., the Mother Force in the Universe and Kûṭastha, the Father, have both been lost in the "Kriyār para avasthā." I, too, with my human consciousness, got lost. But, due to

Divine Grace, I have again been awakened into the Supreme Consciousness.

Kabīr deoyal hāṛkā, māste bāñdhā ān
Khaṛ khaṛ tā pāyā nahi, deoyalkā sahi dān. ***27.***

Kabīr says: "Our body is a temple of bones bound by flesh and within this temple there is God. And yet I could not find Him here due to absence of instructions from the Sadguru."

Note: Without initiation and instruction from the Sadguru the Divine cannot be realized, although He is within us.

Kabīr deoyal ḍhahi paṛā, iṭ bhayi saykor
Citerā cuni cuni gayā, milā nā duji dor. ***28.***

Kabīr says: "The temple has been in ruins and the bricks (i.e. veins) lie scattered here and there (i.e., they have been relaxed; they have lost their tightness). The Kûṭastha has devoured them up completely. And yet I cannot find out the door to the Divine."

Note: Without the Sadguru's Grace even hard spiritual exercises cannot lead one to the Divine. Such exercises without Grace only add to physical strain and ruin.

Kabīr Rām Nām jāneo nahi, bemukh ān hi ān
Ki bhūṣā ki kātrā, khāte gayā parāṇ. ***29.***

Kabīr says: "Without realizing the greatness of the Name of Rāma you have been attached to other things. Thus you have wasted your life by taking chaff and bran (i.e., worthless things) and have been able to do nothing."

Note: If we do not attain the "Kriyār para avasthā", our lives are merely wasted in earthly trifles.

Kabīr Rām piyāre choṛike, kare āor ko jāp
Biśyākera putra yo, kahe kon ko bāp. ***30.***

Kabīr says: "What good will come of chanting names other than that of the dearest Rāma (the Divine)? It will be just like being the son of a prostitute who cannot call anybody his father."

Note: Kriyā is the surest way to meet our Divine Father within us. To be attached to other worldly objects is to deviate from God.

Kabīr yinha Hari ki corī kari, gaye Nām guṇ bhuli
Te Bidhine bāduṛ raco, rahe ūrdvamukh jhuli. ***31.***

Kabīr says: "He who has forgotten the virtues of the Name of Hari (the Divine) because he has stolen Him, is made like a bat by God, and hangs with face upwards."

Note: He who does not practice Kriyās is like one who has misappropriated the Divine, because he is not doing justice to Him. Such a man is constantly full of earthly desires and prays to Heaven for such satisfaction.

Kabīr Rām Nām jānio nahi, bāṇī binaṭhi mūl
Hari tyaji ihāi rahi gayā, anta parimukh dhūl. ***32.***

Kabīr says: "You have not taken the Name of Rāma (the Lord). You, therefore, did not reach the source of words. Since you stay in this world without realizing Hari (the Lord), dust will cover your mouth after death."

Note: 'Bināṭhi' is a stick burning at two ends. The human body has the fire of lust and other kinds of earthly attachment at the lower end and the Divine Fire within the head. If human beings have no realization of this Divine Fire in the 'Kriyār para avasthā", their death will merely mean the destruction of bodies without any taste of Supreme Realization.

Kabīr Rām Nām jānio nahi, lāgi moṭi khoṛi
Kāyā hañṛi kāṭh ki, nā oha caṛe bahori. ***33.***

Kabīr says: "Without knowing the Name of Rāma, you have stuck to the body which is like a thick log of wood. But there, too, you could not climb the wooden vessel, viz., your body."

Note: Without climbing to the top of your body, i.e., without reaching the "Kriyār para avasthā", you cannot hope to have liberated consciousness.

Kabīr Rām Nām jānio nahi, cukeo abki ghāt
Māṭi milan kuñhāṛ ki ghani sahegā lāt. ***34.***

Kabīr says: "You have wasted your life without knowing the Name of Rāma. The potter prepares the clay with the help of his legs and does not leave off till it becomes fit for use in making utensils. But you have not tried to make your body a fit medium for Self-Realization."

Note: The devotee should go on practicing Kriyās till he reaches the Supreme Realization in the "Kriyār para avasthā."

Kabīr eha samsār me, ghanā manikh matahīn
Rām Nām jānīo nahi, aye buṛpāpā din. ***35.***

Kabīr says that many persons in this world are lacking in duties instructed by the Scriptures. They do not take the Name of Rāma either. Hence they are easily weakened by old age.

Note: The Name of Rāma here stands for the "Kriyār para avasthā." Most persons do not practice the Kriyās (duties sanctioned by the Scriptures); hence it is impossible for them to reach the "Kriyār para avasthā." So they are easily overtaken by mortality.

Kabīr kahe kiyā tum āike, kahe karoge yāy
Itke bhaye na uoke, cale janma jaharāy. ***36.***

Kabīr says: "What have you done after coming to this world? And what can you do after this life? You have done nothing in this world, nor have you done anything for your life after death. Hence your life has been wasted in vain."

Note: Practicing Kriyās in earthly life is a preparation for the "Kriyār para avasthā" which is the life eternal. Human life, therefore, should be properly utilized in practicing Kriyās.

Kabīr ek Hari ki bhakti binu, dhrk jīvan samsār
Dhūākā dhaur har yyo, yāt na lāge bār. ***37.***

Kabīr says: "It is useless to live in this world without taking the Name of Hari (the Lord). As the tip of the plow does not delay in piercing the earth, so also you will enter death in no time."

Note: A life without Divine Consciousness is worse than death.

Kabīr jagat māha man rāñcia, jhuñṭe kul ki lāj
Tan binaśe kul binase, raṭe na Rām jāhāj. ***38.***

Kabīr says: "You have concentrated your mind in the worldly objects and in family pride. But your family, like your body, will not last long. You have not taken shelter in the ship of the Name of Rāma (which would carry you across the ocean of earthly attachment)."

Note: Unless one takes shelter in the Name of Rāma i.e., unless one practices Kriyā, one only proceeds towards mortality.

Kabīr eha tan kāñcā kumbha hāy, coṭ lāge phuṭi yāy
Ekai Harike Nām binu, jab tab jīu jahaṛāy. ***39.***

Kabīr says: "This (human) body is like a pitcher made of clay which has not yet been dried properly. Without the Name of Hari a man may die any moment.."

Note: Unless "Kriyār para avasthā" has been reached, human life can only be a prey to earthly ravages.

Kabīr eha tan kāñcā kumbha hāy, liye ki ratna hāy sāth
Ṭhabkā lāgā phuṭi gayā, kachu nahi āyā hāth. ***40.***

Kabīr says: "You carry a body which is nothing but a pitcher of clay. Any moment it may be broken. What, then, will be your asset?"

Note: Without spiritual enlightenment a mere biological existence is nothing.

Kabīr eha tan kāñcā kumbha hāy, mūṛha kane biśvas
Kahe Kabīr bicārike, nahi palakki āś. ***41.***

Kabīr says: "This body is like a pitcher of clay and fools alone depend on it (as something permanent). Kabīr, after careful consideration, says that this body cannot be trusted even for a moment."

Note: Our time should not be wasted in mere physical enjoyments.

Kabīr pani māhañkā budbudā, dekhat gayā bilāy
Yyāyśa hi jīārā yāyegā, din daś ṭhogri lagāy. ***42.***

Kabīr says: "As bubbles in water vanish before your eyes, so also this human life will pass away in no time. You are only moving about for a few days here."

Note: The body is mortal. But the Blessed Consciousness can be attained through Kriyās.

Kabīr eha tan yāt hāy, śake to ṭhor lāgāyo
Rājā Rāṇā sabh gayā, kāhu na rahiyā ṭhāyo. ***43.***

Kabīr says: "The body is fast decaying. Stick to something eternal if you can. Kings and commanders have all passed away from this world; none could stay here for all time."

Note: Since the body is moving towards death, one should try for steadfastness in the "Kriyār para avasthā" as soon as one can.

Kabīr eha tan yāt hāy, śake to bhu bahori
Namgī hāthete gaye, yāke lākh karor. ***44.***

Kabīr says: "Keep back this fast-aging body if you can; for even multi-millionaires have not been able to take a single farthing with themselves at the time of death."

Note: Physical death is inevitable. But we should achieve the immortality of Consciousness through Kriyās.

Kabīr bāsar sukh nahi bayen sukh, nā sukh avapne māha
Yo nar bichure Rām soñ, tinha ko dhūp na chāñha. ***45.***

Kabīr says that people who are forgetful of Rāma (the Divine) have no happiness during day or night. They are not even happy in their dreams. They have neither the Sun nor the shadow (i.e., no happiness on any side).

Note: Without God-contact through the Kriyās, man cannot be really happy.

Kabīr din goñyāyā mufatme, duniyā na lāgi sāṭh
Pāo kulhāṅ māriā, gāphil apne hāth. ***46.***

Kabīr says: "You have spent the day in useless work. This world will not go with you. You have struck your own legs with an axe as it were by your lack of attention to the Divine."

Note: Not to practice Kriyās will mean sheer waste of time.

Kabīr eha tan ban bhayā, karma yo bhayā kulhār
Apne āpu ko kātiā, kahe Kabīr bicār. ***47.***

Kabīr says that this body has been full of forests, and duties are like axes. Kabīr, after due consideration, advises to clear the forests of sins with the axes.

Note: To work for the satisfaction of earthly desires is attachment. Practicing Kriyās is performance of duties without attachment. Kriyāyoga, practiced for a long time, banishes all attachment, all slavery to desires.

Kabīr kūl khoye kūl ubre, kūl rākhe, kūl yāy
Rām akūl kūl meṭiyā, sabhkul gayā bilāy. ***48.***

Kabīr says: "If you destroy the beach, it comes again. If you want to keep it, it moves away. When Rāma will satisfy the beach and the sea, the beach, too, will vanish."

Note: God (the Ātmā) is the reconciliation of all opposites. Once we reach God-contact through Kriyās, we are beyond the reach of all earthly shores.

Kabīr duniyāke dhoñkhe muyā, calā yo kul ki kāṇ
Tab kā ko kul lājasi, yay lay dhare masān. ***49.***

Kabīr says: "Everybody is deceived by the illusion of the world. Everybody is proceeding according to family traditions and by hearsay. At the time of death, however, these will not save your shame."

Note: Most people are slaves to a false sense of family prestige and idle talks. But these are great obstacles on the path of the Divine.

Kabīr kul karaṇīke kāraṇe, hamsā cale bigoy
Tab ka ko kul lājasi, yab cāri caraṇkā hoy. **50.**

Kabīr says: "You have not been born for showing off family prestige. When the Swan (the Soul) leaves your body, the dead body will be carried to the ground of cremation on the shoulders of four persons. Who will feel the family pride or shame at that time?"

Note: Family pride or such other attachment will not do us any good.

Kabīr kul karaṇīke kārane hoye rahā nal sūm
Tab ka ko kul lājasi, yab Yam dhūmā dhūm. **51.**

Kabīr says: "People become miserly, for they think money must needs be saved for maintaining traditional family expenditure. But when the God of death will come to overtake them with great ceremony, who will think of the family prestige?"

Note: People often worship God for the sake of custom and formality. Real worship would come from the heart and would lead them to the practice of Kriyāyoga.

Kabīr kul karaṇī ki pāgrī, küp kaṭhor tā māhi
Bāñci cala so ubrā, nahi to buṛā tāhi. **52.**

Kabīr says that the pitcher of family duties remains immersed in a well. If it is raised from the well, it gets saved; otherwise it becomes drowned.

Note: This world is like a well and work for the fulfillment of earthly desires is like a pitcher. He who is obsessed with worldly attachment gets drowned in the well. But he who practices Kriyā gets saved and rises upwards into the life eternal.

Kabīr yetā ḍar hāy jāt ki, tetā Hari ki hoy
Dhol damāmā dei cale, calā na pakṛe koy. **53.**

Kabīr says: "Do you fear God so much as you fear the rules of caste and community? If you would be so very God-fearing, people would be eager to follow you with drums and bugles, but they would not be able to catch you."

Note: Pride and prejudice associated with noble birth, e.g., may prevent a person from mixing with a Saintly person of lower birth. Family ties and such other sentiments often stand in the way of a man's doing what is right. But if a man is God-fearing, he will always hesitate to commit anything wrong.

Kabīr keval Rām ko, tu mati choṛe ot
Nāto aharla ghawna bikhe, ghani sahegā coṭ. ***54.***

Kabīr says: "Rāma alone is your shelter. Do not abandon his protection. If you divert your attention to anything else, you will have to suffer the pangs of repeated births and deaths."

Note: The "kevala karma" or work for the liberation of the soul is the Kriyāyoga. If one does not practice Kriyās, one will have to be born again and again and suffer untold misery.

Kabīr keval Rām kahu, sujagari bā jhāri
Kul baṛai buṛasī, bhārī parasi māri. ***55.***

Kabīr says: "Coming to this beautiful world, do your duties to Rāma (the Lord). You will then conquer your family traditions and pride and kill a very important neighbor."

Note: Kriyā will gradually make us conquer pride prejudice. It will also make the Jīvātmā, the human consciousness, merge into the Paramātmā or the Divine. This merging has been described by Kabīr as the death of a near neighbor.

Kabīr kāyā mañjan kyā kare, kapṛā dhoyan khoy
ujal bhaye na chuṭasi, yo man mail na khoy. ***56.***

Kabīr says: "What would you do by cleansing your body and washing your clothes? The dirt of the mind will not be removed by merely washing the body, and unless the mind is purified, the required state of consciousness will not be attained."

Note: The mind can be pure only by meditation on the Divine, and for such meditation Kriyāyoga is essential.

Kabīr ujal pekhe kāpṛā, pān supāri khāy
Ek Harike Nām binu, bāñdhā yampur yāy. ***57.***

Kabīr says: "People are moving about like fashionable gentlemen with clean garments, their mouths full of betel-leaves and nuts. But when he will have to voyage to the land of death, tied hands and feet, none of his near and dear ones will be of any help to him. His only asset at that time will be the Name of the Lord."

Note: "Kriyār para avasthā" is the only final asset to the human soul, liberating it as it does from the ties of earthly attachment.

Kabīr ḍar poñṭeṅ pāg soñ, mati mayli hoy yāy
Pāg becāri kyā kare, yau śir nahi māṭi khāy. ***58.***

Kabīr says: "If the mind remains constantly engaged in tightening the head-dress, it will have no time to cleanse itself of impurities. The turban will not save him from being transformed into the dust after death."

Note: Nothing else but God-contact through Kriyās can save man from bondage.

Kabīr mandil māhi pauṙte, parimal ang lagāy
Chatrapatike rākhme, gadhā loṭe yāy. ***59.***

Kabīr says: "The body has been purified and made fragrant due to its stay in the temple and even the ass has laid itself prostrate at the feet of the King."

Note: Due to contact with the Divine through Kriyāyoga, the body becomes pure. All human beings lacking in Divine consciousness may be considered fools (asses). But Kriyā links them up with the Kûṭastha and they can gradually attain "Kriyār para avasthā."

Kabīr gaukhan māhi pauṙte parimal ang lagāy
Svapnā sama dekhat rahe, gayā so bahuri bilāy. ***60.***

Kabīr says: "While performing with my tongue some practices given by the Master (the Guru), I had attained purity of my limbs. I was having visions as in a dream, but now they have disappeared."

Note: While practicing Kriyās with the tongue, the devotee experiences innumerable visions in the Kûṭastha. But the very same vision does not generally recur.

Kabīr khāsāmal pahiñte, khāte nāgar pān
Tebhi hote mānabī karte bahut gumān. ***61.***

Kabīr says: "Men wear clean clothes, chew betels and show themselves off with pride. They always search out other people's faults, although they are indifferent to those of themselves. And yet such people call themselves men."

Note: People engaged in fashionable artificialities are far away from God.

Kabīr jangal ḍheri rākh ki, upar ghās patang
Tebhi hoye mānavī, karte rang berang. ***62.***

Kabīr says: "A forest has developed on the stack of ashes and rubbish, where grass has grown and insects move about. Such is ordinary human life full of variegated colors."

Note: This body is nothing but ashes, because everybody will be burnt to ashes after death. Even when we have so much of earthly affection.

Kabīr merā sangī koi nahi, sabhe sāranthī loy
Man paratīm na upje, jīu biśrām na hoy. ***63.***

Kabīr says: "I have no companion. Even if I have some, they all would like to be my guides. Since the mind has no faith in them, it becomes restless."

Note: In the "Kriyār para avasthā" the devotee becomes one with the Divine and therefore he becomes One without a second. But before he attains to that stage, different and conflicting emotions lead him this way and that, making his mind restless all the while. Kriyā is the surest method to control the erring mind and concentrate it in the Divine.

Kabīr thal carantā mirgala, ek yo bedhā soha
Ham to pāthi basi rahā, pheri karegā kaunhā? ***64.***

Kabīr says: "The deer was moving about. He who has pierced him is myself. I, a passer-by, have now been sitting idle. Who, then, will do the selling?"

Note: The human body is the deer. It is generally restless, but it can be quiet when pierced by the Ātmā (the self) through Prāṇāyāma. The human consciousness is like a restless traveller, but through practices in Kriyās it can be concentrated in the Divine till at last it merges in Supreme Consciousness in the "Kriyār para avasthā."

Kabīr it ghar ut ghar onā, banijan āye hāṭ
Karma phirānā becike caliye apni bāṭ. ***65.***

Kabīr says: "Leaving my own room I have come to another's, just as traders go over to the marketplace for transaction of business. After their work, however, they return to their own houses."

Note: We are like traders who have come to human bodies for suffering the fruits of our work in previous births. When our duties will be finished here, we shall go back to God who is our home. Our reaching the "Kriyār para avasthā" through prolonged practices of Kriyās is our home-coming.

Kabīr mārag upar dauṃā, sukh nidari nā śoy
Parā parāye deśrā, ochi ṭhor na khoy. ***66.***

Kabīr says: "You will have to rush along the road. Do not waste time in idle sleep; for that land is beyond every other country. May you not lose that in fruitless sleep!"

Note: Through practices in Kriyās we will have to rush along the Suṣumnā, that subtle passage within the spinal cord, which leads us to the Divine within the head. The Sahasrāra, the thousand-petalled lotus within the head, is the main seat of God in the human body. To reach that sacred zone through Prāṇāyāma is our aim. Without wasting our time in idleness we should try to reach that place by all means. When our consciousness is settled there, we have absolute Bliss in the "Kriyār para avasthā."

Kabīr nāo yo jhajhri, kurso kheyoān hār
Haluke haluke tari gaye, buṛe yinha śir bhār. ***67.***

Kabīr says: "The boat that is there is full of holes. The oar, too, does not work well. Those who were light will somehow reach the shore, but the heavy-headed ones will be drowned."

Note: The body is like a boat having as many as nine holes (viz., the mouth, the two nostrils, the two eyes, the two ears, the penis and the anus), conducted by an evil mind. Those who are slightly bad will, through prolonged practice of Kriyās, reach the Divine Consciousness with some difficulty. But men, whose heads are heavily filled with bad motives, will be destroyed. The nine holes or doors to the body are the organs through which we establish contact with the outside world and get into earthly attachment. Through Kriyās, these contacts are gradually turned inwards, to the Divine.

Kabīr Rām kahante khijhi mare, kuśrī h gali yāy
Śukar hoyeke āo tare, nāk buṛante khāy. ***68.***

Kabīr says: "Those who have great distaste for the Name of Rāma, become ugly and melt away. Like hogs they feed by dipping their nose."

Note: Those who are averse to Kriyās, have to suffer from physical ills and mental restlessness. Their minds constantly remain engaged in the dirty things of life, just like boars who roll in the mire.

Kabīr yā mat sā mat tāmta, tā mat tāo na sāo
Rām binā sab bharm haāy, Rājā Rāṇā Rāo. ***69.***

Kabīr says: "The worldly customs and traditions are generally established by kings and princes. But all these, when they do not lead to Rāma (the Divine), are full of errors."

Note: Kriyā is the method of knowing our Lord. Rules and regulations which deviate the mind from the Kriyā are no proper guides in life.

Kabīr eha pur pāṭan deśoā, pānc cor dās doyār
Man Rājā gaṁme lahe, sumiri lehu kartār. ***70.***

Kabīr says: "This body is like a covered space having ten doors and five thieves in it. It is like a castle whereof the mind is the king. Go on remembering the Lord in such circumstances."

Note: The five thieves in the body are our five senses (viz., vision, hearing, smell, taste and touch) which engage our mind with outward objects and thus deviate it from the Divine. The ten doors are the two eyes, the two ears, the two nostrils, the mouth, the penis the anus and the subtlest opening at the crest of the head – the 'Brahma-randhra' or hole of the Divine, which generally remains closed but opens up through the Kriyās. While nine gates of the body establish contact with the outside world, the tenth gate within the head leads us to liberation. The soul of the Yogī leaves the body at the time of death through this tenth gate. But the mind, through Kriyās, must always remain engaged in the Divine before we hope to open this tenth gate.

Kabīr pipri lunāy phul binu, kul binu lunāy na yāy
Ekā ekī mānasā, dhāñpā dinho āy. ***71.***

Kabīr says: "A peepul tree is visible without flowers, and that is nothing but Kula-kuṇḍalinī. The mind, when concentrated in that, attains to 'Samādhi' (complete absorption in the Divine)."

Note: The 'Kula-kuṇḍalinī' is the latent Divine Energy in the human body at the very base of the 'Suṣumnā'. By means of Kriyāyoga this Energy rises up through the spinal cord and gets merged in the Supreme Self within the head.

Kabīr myay to hi bhaurā barjiā, ban ban bāsan lehu
Āṭkegā koi bel so, talphi talphi jīu lehu. ***72.***

Kabīr says: "My mind is like a black bee which has been roaming about in the forest of life. 'O my mind! do not get attached to transitory things. You might get entangled in some desire, which, like a creeper entangling the wings of a black bee, will destroy you outright."

Note: A restless mind, not restrained by Kriyās will only bring disaster.

Kabīr bejhā bhaun rathā leta kalihu ko bās
So to bhaunrā uṛi gayā, choṛi bāri ki āś. ***73.***

Kabīr says: "The black bee, mind, confined within the body, used to smell the buds (i.e., earthly desires). Now it has flown away, abandoning the expectation of water (i.e.,honey)."

Note: The mind, in order to be liberated from petty earthly desires, will have to be united with the Divine through Kriyās.

Kabīr maṇik moti kāñkrā, Nām na hosi koy
Yyāsā sāheb sei le, duno dinkā hoy. ***74.***

Kabīr says: "Jewels and pearls are but as stones. They are not at all valuable like the sacred Name of God. Serve such a Master (viz., God) who is able to provide for you in this life as well as in the hereafter."

Note: To attain "Kriyār para avasthā" is the highest aim of human life. One who has reached this state of Transcendent Consciousness, is free from all kinds of fear and anxiety.

Kabīr bār bār to so kaha, śunre manuā nīc
Baṇijāreke bayel yo, peṛe hi māhi mic. ***75.***

Kabīr says: "O base mind! if you do not pay heed to what I repeatedly tell you, you will be destroyed like a trader's bullock who was put to death by simply moving about in different countries on errands of his trading master."

Note: Unless we reach the "Kriyār para avasthā", we shall have to be born on this earth again. This is the result of serving Mammon instead of the Divine.

Kabīr baṇijāreke bayel yeño, ṭāñṛā utrā yāy
E kahuke dunā bhaye, ek cale mul gañoyāy. ***76.***

Kabīr says: "When the two bundles of a trader's bullock hanging from both sides of his back get mixed up, both of them drop down because of too much weight. So also, we should not confuse the material with the spiritual lest we lose both."

Note: Material attachment stands in the way of the liberation of our soul.

Kabīr dariā kṣārā deha hāy, cārived tehi māhi
Koi Sant vivekī bāñci hāy, nā tau buṛā tāhi. ***77.***

Kabīr says: "This body may be likened to an Ocean of salt waters. And although even the four Vedas (i.e., Self-knowledge) are there within the body, most people have been immersed in the saline water, and only a few conscientious Saints are living."

Note: Only those who have reached the 'Kriyār para avasthā' are actually living, for it is they who have tasted of the Life Eternal. The rest of the human beings remain immersed in endless desires from which only spiritual practices (Kriyās) under the instruction of a Sadguru can raise them up.

Kabīr purkhanī nyāyārā sabhante, sabhe kahe sujh māhi
Upajat binu sat ei sandā, āye thīr koi nāhi ***78.***

Kabīr says: "The Self is distinct from everything else, and all (the sages) tell us to look into our own selves. But the sight of so many births and deaths makes men restless (because they doubt the concept of immortality of the soul)."

Note: Kriyā is the gatepass to the inner world where one can realize the ultimate identity of the limited human self with the Self Supreme. Without Self-Realization it is not possible to fathom the mystery of births and deaths.

Kabīr pāñc tattva kā putrā, tā maha pañchī paun
Rahane kā ācrāy giṇo, yāt ācambhā kaun. ***79.***

Kabīr says: "There is a bird within this doll of five elements (i.e., the body which is composed of earth, water, fire, air, space). That the bird stays there at all is strange. There is nothing strange about its flight."

Note: The bird is the soul within the body. People generally wonder at death which is the passing away of the soul, the immortal part, from the body. But is it not more strange that something immortal has taken habitation within this mortal frame?

Kabīr pāñco ke madhime, phiri dhare śarir
Yo pāñcko baśī kare, soi lāgad tīr. ***80.***

Kabīr says: "Under the influence of the five elements men have to be born again and again. But he who can conquer these elements, reaches the shore."

Note: Through Kriyās we can reach beyond the sense-impression of material life and enjoy Divine Bliss.

Kabīr cet nihārā cetiyā, ar yo ceto yāy
Kahe Kabīr ceto nahi, bahuri bahuri pachtāy. ***81.***

Kabīr says: "Offer your heart to Him who gives you consciousness. If you do not do that, you will have to be born and die time and again."

Note: We shall have to surrender ourselves to the Supreme Self through Kriyās. Then, and then alone, we shall be the inheritors of Eternity.

Kabīr bhay binu bhāv na upje, bhay binu hoy na Prīti
Yab hi darśo bhay gai, tab meṭi sakal ras rīti. ***82.***

Kabīr says: "Without fear there cannot be any love or union. When the fear is dispelled, idle pleasures also have an end."

Note: Unless there would be fear of death, men would not generally try to liberate their souls. Spiritualism, therefore, often starts in fear. Then, through practices in Kriyās, people try to be united with the deathless Reality. Once, however, the supreme state of consciousness is reached, earthly joys and sorrows cease to have any appreciable influence on man.

Kabīr bhay soñ sabhi bhakti kare, bhayte pujā hoy
Bhay māre eha jīu ko, binu bhay kāj na koy. ***83.***

Kabīr says: "It is out of fear that people offer devotion and worship. Nobody would do anything excepting out of this fear. It is fear again which kills a man."

Note: The Guru has asked the disciple to practice Kriyā, and the disciple often does it for fear, lest there should be any harm without it.

Kabīr dar pāraś dar Param Guru, ḍar karaṇī ḍar sār
Dartā raha so ubre, gāphīl khāyā mār. ***84.***

Kabīr says: "Fear is the touchstone; fear is the great Guru; fear is the root and essence of work. He who has no fear for God, will be destroyed."

Note: A God-fearing soul will practice Kriyās and will ultimately, be saved.

Kabīr khāli mili khāli bhayā, bahut kiyā bakvād
Bāñjhaha lāoye pālnā, tāme kon saovād. ***85.***

Kabīr says: "You have spent your time uselessly and have been through much idle talk. Like a childless mother who rocks the cradle in the expectation of a child to be born, the idle talker also goes on giving out his comments on so many things."

Note: If anybody does not have realization of the Divine and yet delivers lectures on spiritual matters, his can only be idle talks signifying nothing.

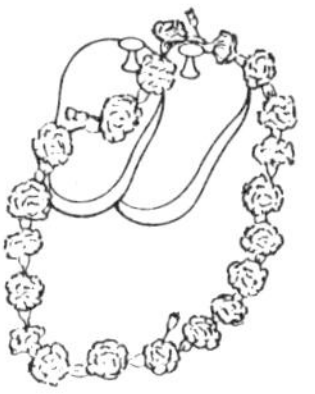

EDITIONS PUBLISHED BY AMRITA FOUNDATION, INC.

The original, unchanged writings of
Paramhansa (Swami) Yogananda

The Second Coming of Christ, Vol.1
The Second Coming of Christ, Vol.2
The Second Coming of Christ, Vol.3

The Sermon on the Mount (Interpretations of)

Metaphysical Meditations (1932 First Edition)
Divine Perceptions – Interpretations of
Genesis, Revelation and the Bhagavad-Gita
PRAECEPTA® Lessons of Paramhansa Yogananda

The original, unchanged writings of Swami Yogananda Giri
and Swami Dhirananda Giri, Associate (Dr. Basu Kumar Bagchi)

The Science of Religion (1920 First Edition)
Psychological Chart (1921 First Edition)
Songs of the Soul (1923 First Edition)
Scientific Healing Affirmations (1924 First Edition)
Whispers From Eternity (1929 First Edition)
PRAECEPTA® BOOK (1923 First Edition)

The original, unchanged writings of Swami Dhirananda
(Dr. Basu Kumar Bagchi)

Philosophical Insights (1925 First Edition)
Glimpses of Light (1929 First Edition)
Raja Yoga Series (1929 First Edition)

The Hound of Heaven by Francis Thompson
(An early 1900's English edition)

Yogiraj Shri Shri Lahiri Mahashay by J.C. Bhattacharya
(1964 First Edition)

Kabīr: In the Light of Kriyayoga by J.C. Bhattacharya
(1974 First Edition)